Reading the Nineteenth-Century Medical Journal

This book explores medical and health periodicals of the nineteenth century: their contemporary significance, their readership, and how historians have approached them as objects of study.

From debates about women doctors in lesser-known titles such as the *Medical Mirror*, to the formation of professional medical communities within French and Portuguese periodicals, the contributors to this volume highlight the multi-faceted nature of these publications as well as their uses to the historian. Medical periodicals – far from being the preserve of doctors and nurses – were also read by the general public. Thus, the contributions collected here will be of interest not only to the historian of medicine, but also to those interested in nineteenth-century periodical culture more broadly.

The chapters in this book were originally published as a special issue of the journal *Media History*.

Sally Frampton is Humanities and Healthcare Fellow at the University of Oxford, UK. Her publications have focused on the history of surgery and the development of medical journalism in the nineteenth century, and include her monograph *Belly-Rippers, Surgical Innovation and the Ovariotomy Controversy* (2018).

Jennifer Wallis is Medical Humanities Teaching Fellow and Lecturer in the History of Science and Medicine at Imperial College London, UK. Her publications include *Investigating the Body in the Victorian Asylum: Doctors, Patients, and Practices* (2017) and the co-authored volume *Anxious Times: Medicine and Modernity in Nineteenth-Century Britain* (2019).

Reading the Nineteenth-Century Medical Journal

Edited by
Sally Frampton and Jennifer Wallis

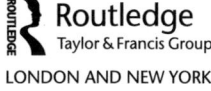

Routledge
Taylor & Francis Group

LONDON AND NEW YORK

First published 2021
by Routledge
2 Park Square, Milton Park, Abingdon, Oxon OX14 4RN

and by Routledge
52 Vanderbilt Avenue, New York, NY 10017

Routledge is an imprint of the Taylor & Francis Group, an informa business

British Library Cataloguing in Publication Data
A catalogue record for this book is available from the British Library

ISBN 13: 978-0-367-64326-3

Typeset in MyriadPro
by Newgen Publishing UK

Publisher's Note
The publisher accepts responsibility for any inconsistencies that may have arisen during
the conversion of this book from journal articles to book chapters, namely the inclusion of
journal terminology.

Disclaimer
Every effort has been made to contact copyright holders for their permission to reprint
material in this book. The publishers would be grateful to hear from any copyright holder
who is not here acknowledged and will undertake to rectify any errors or omissions in future
editions of this book.

Contents

Citation Information

The chapters in this book were originally published in *Media History*, volume 25, issue 1 (2019). When citing this material, please use the original page numbering for each article, as follows:

Introduction

Reading Medicine and Health in Periodicals
Sally Frampton and Jennifer Wallis
Media History, volume 25, issue 1 (2019), pp. 1–5

Chapter 1

The 'Medical-Women Question' and the Multivocality of the Victorian Medical Press, 1869–1900
Alison Moulds
Media History, volume 25, issue 1 (2019), pp. 6–22

Chapter 2

Shaping Doctors and Society: The Portuguese Medical Press (1880–1926)
Ana Carneiro, Teresa Salomé Mota and Isabel Amaral
Media History, volume 25, issue 1 (2019), pp. 23–50

Chapter 3

Reading Photography in French Nineteenth Century Journals
Beatriz Pichel
Media History, volume 25, issue 1 (2019), pp. 51–69

Chapter 4

'Bicycle-Face' and 'Lawn Tennis' Girls: Debating girls' health in late nineteenth- and early twentieth-century British periodicals
Hilary Marland
Media History, volume 25, issue 1 (2019), pp. 70–84

Chapter 5

Using Digitised Medical Journals in a Cross European Project on Addiction History
Alex Mold and Virginia Berridge
Media History, volume 25, issue 1 (2019), pp. 85–99

For any permission-related enquiries please visit:
www.tandfonline.com/page/help/permissions

Notes on Contributors

Isabel Amaral, Faculty of Science and Technology – DCSA and CIUHCT, NOVA New University of Lisbon, Campus de Caparica, Portugal.

Virginia Berridge, London School of Hygiene and Tropical Medicine, London, UK.

Ana Carneiro, Faculty of Science and Technology – DCSA and CIUHCT, NOVA New University of Lisbon, Campus de Caparica, Caparica, Portugal.

Sally Frampton, Faculty of History, University of Oxford, UK.

Hilary Marland, Department of History, University of Warwick, Coventry, UK.

Alex Mold, London School of Hygiene and Tropical Medicine, London, UK.

Teresa Salomé Mota, Geologist, former researcher in the CIUHCT, University of Lisbon, Portugal.

Alison Moulds, Independent Scholar, former researcher at the Faculty of English Language and Literature, University of Oxford, UK, and the Department of Humanities, University of Roehampton, UK.

Beatriz Pichel, Photographic History Research Centre, De Montfort University, Leicester, UK.

Jennifer Wallis, Faculty of Medicine, Imperial College London, UK.

INTRODUCTION
READING MEDICINE AND HEALTH IN PERIODICALS

Sally Frampton and Jennifer Wallis

This special issue of Media History, *arising from a workshop on nineteenth-century medical and health periodicals, aims to explore both the contemporary significance and readership of these periodicals, but also how their study has been approached by historians. We discuss existing work on medical periodicals—considering how these publications have been studied by literary and historical scholars—and how our understanding and use of them has developed in an era of digitisation. Finally, we examine how the contributors to this volume each highlight important issues in terms of the interpretation, reading, and materiality of medical and health periodicals.*

In May 2015 the Oxford University-based projects Constructing Scientific Communities and Diseases of Modern Life ran a joint workshop, 'Working with Nineteenth-Century Medical and Health Periodicals'. The purpose of the workshop was to bring together historians and literary scholars working closely with the vast range of medical and health-related periodicals which materialised in the nineteenth century. We wanted to cast wide questions with which we ourselves were getting to grips with throughout the two projects. Which medical periodicals had so far eluded historical scrutiny? How might their significance be defined? How were changing methodologies and practices, particularly digitisation, affecting medical historians in their approaches to periodicals? The response to our call for papers exceeded expectations, and the articles in this special issue showcase the diverse scholarly work currently being undertaken, expansive in both its geographical and methodological scope. The papers presented here, focusing largely on the late nineteenth and early twentieth centuries, reflect the contemporary increase in the number of medical and health periodicals on the market, the growth of medical specialisation, and the expansion of the periodical-reading public from the latter half of the nineteenth century.[1] They build upon a pre-existing but relatively small pool of historical work on medical periodicals. In the British context, the classic text in the field is the edited volume by W.F Bynum, Stephen Lock, and Roy Porter, *Medical Journals and Medical Knowledge: Historical Essays* (1992), which makes valuable in-roads into disentangling the complex historical world of medical periodicals, where, from the late eighteenth century, countless titles arose, succeeded, failed, merged, split or faded away; most have left little in the way of significant clues about their production or readership. Nonetheless the volume was one of the first forays into the history of medical journalism which recognised the sheer scale of the medical periodical market, and particularly its expansion during the nineteenth century, during which an estimated 479 medical journals were established in Britain.[2] Bynum, Lock, and Porter also acknowledged (and critiqued) the apparent separation between historians of medicine and those of periodicals; 'what this volume abundantly shows are the pitfalls of such arbitrary separations of the medium from the message', they wrote.[3]

It is a separation that has led to two somewhat discrete historiographical narratives; Victorian literature scholars have more assiduously explored the role of general periodicals in shaping understandings of health and medicine. Work by Cynthia Ellen Patton and Claire Furlong for example, on health advice columns in lay publications *Girls' Own Paper* (Patton) and *Reynold's Miscellany* and the *Family Herald* (Furlong), have elucidated the relationship between health, patient agency, and the press in ways that look beyond the major medical periodicals.[4] Historians of medicine on the other hand, have tended to focus on the emergence and impact of the weekly medical periodical in the early nineteenth century and in particular that most recognisable of titles, the *Lancet*, begun in 1823 by general practitioner Thomas Wakley as a means of opening up the corrupt and closeted world of the medical elite, and who through the pages of his periodical widely disseminated hospital lectures as well as the latest medical news and gossip. Taking heed of Bynum's call to recognise both content and form, in recent years, Brittany Pladek and Michael Brown have explored the broader influences of popular and political journalism respectively on the *Lancet*, and the interplay between the periodical's cost, frequency, and literary style.[5] This has been augmented by Carin Berkowitz's examination of medical journalism in early nineteenth-century Britain, in particular the relationships between the *Lancet* and 'rival' titles such as the *London Medical Gazette* and the medico-political ideologies of those periodicals and their users.[6]

That medical historians often continue to focus on the *Lancet* and its immediate contemporaries is, perhaps, not surprising given the seismic impact that the periodical had, dramatically challenging the norms of medical professional culture. Its presence also continues to be felt today, as Britain's leading medical journal.[7] The disproportionate focus upon it mirrors that within nineteenth-century scholarship upon publications such as *The Times*, as discussed by Andrew Hobbs. But as Hobbs puts it, 'longevity in journalism should not be confused with significance'.[8] When we begin to look beyond the horizons of these big names—seminal though they were—we find myriad other periodicals that, despite their limited life span, also need to be assimilated into any thorough account of the nineteenth-century medical press, including those publications that have proved less attractive in digitisation ventures or which do not have obvious contemporary resonance. The 'Working with Nineteenth-Century Medical and Health Periodicals' workshop aimed to address these issues head-on, bringing together historians of medicine with historians of the periodical press to explore how the two fields could be best synthesised—sharing our findings and comparing our methodologies. Prominent in our discussion was the issue of digitisation. The nineteenth century-scholar, in particular, has benefited from digitisation projects such as ProQuest's British Periodicals and the British Library's 19th Century Newspapers Database, and although many of us may not think of ourselves as 'digital historians' it is increasingly difficult to reject that designation if we belong to an institution with access to digital resources.[9] Large-scale digitisation programmes such as that undertaken by the Medical Heritage Library, a collaborative endeavour between medical libraries, of which UK-based institutions have played a major part, mean that an ever growing storehouse of digitised material is available to medical historians, some of whom have already begun to examine the implications, possibilities, and challenges for the field of working with 'Big Data'.[10] Using a combination of traditional and digital research can be enormously profitable. But for all its benefits, the increasing proliferation of digitised content has also led to notes of caution regarding its use, apparent in some of the questions raised in this issue.

The abundance of medical periodical literature that emerged in the nineteenth century can make the analysis of them a task of some magnitude. But as Alison Moulds shows in her examination of 'the medical-women question' in the nineteenth-century British medical press in this issue, even within the scope of one periodical, attempting to locate a key message or perspective can be problematic, and opinions and viewpoints were constantly in flux. Moulds uncovers a 'multiplicity of voices', some in favour of the study and practice of medicine by women and some staunchly opposed. The multiple voices that she finds—such as the women who wrote to the *Lancet* to protest against the possibility of 'lady doctors'—tell us as much about contemporary reading practices as they do professional medical attitudes towards women doctors, with the periodical having reach beyond the confines of the qualified, male, doctor.

Exploring another aspect to the intersection between periodical culture and professional groupings, Ana Carneiro, Isabel Amaral and Teresa Salomé Mota edge us into the twentieth century with their in-depth exploration of the Portuguese medical press, which gives geographical nuance to a medical periodical culture often read solely through developments in Northern Europe and America. The manner in which a 'medical press' emerges as an influential entity in a particular locale is a phenomenon that requires explication. The large number of medical periodicals that began in Portugal between 1880 and 1926, Carneiro et al show, enacted doctors' scientific and professional, as well as social and cultural, aspirations. Moreover, such periodicals were intended to have an impact beyond the boundaries of the medical profession, in particular to align the public's health with the values of Portugal's new republican regime, and thus they should be read within a political frame of reference.

Beatriz Pichel's article further elucidates the need for medical periodicals to be understood in contexts beyond the history of medicine. Pichel navigates through the French medical press via photography—an element of nineteenth-century printed matter that is often lost in the digitisation process. Focusing on periodicals that arose from the field of psychology, Pichel highlights the diverse ways photography was put to work within different titles, dependent on the school of psychology the periodical adhered to, and which saw differing strategies employed to meet the varying expectations and needs of editors, authors, and readers. By employing a photographic history approach, Pichel also identifies an interplay between medical and theatrical literature, which engendered connections and crossover between scientific and popular audiences.

Such connections are also visible in Hilary Marland's examination of debates around girls' health at the turn of the century. As Marland shows, a range of popular health and lay periodicals facilitated these debates, which often involved multiple actors from both within and outside of the medical profession. The periodicals that Marland cites, such as *Good Health*, neither entirely generalist nor strictly medical, are particularly important in demonstrating the complexities and proliferation of periodical culture during this era: the increasing amount of literature written by doctors but targeted at a lay audience suggests that no easy distinction between professional medical and popular health discourse can be made.

The plethora and diversity of medical and health periodicals available in the late nineteenth and early twentieth centuries, some of it now available through digitisation, mean it is easy to be carried away by the wealth of material almost literally at one's finger-tips—pages and pages of hits returned via a simple word search. But digital material cannot simply replace the physical, as Alex Mold and Virginia Berridge highlight in their article. One of the most fruitful areas for research using digital materials is the analysis of language—tracking the changing usage of words over time, or using search tools to uncover common relationships between words—and Mold and Berridge set out to chart how the language used in connection with habitual drug, alcohol, or tobacco use has changed since the mid-nineteenth century. Their article recounts the challenges that they faced in seeking to compare language use across a number of countries including Italy, Austria, Poland and the UK. They reach important new conclusions, finding linguistic and conceptual variations, as well as commonalities, in the ways different countries framed alcohol and addiction. But their article also highlights the difficulty of relying too heavily upon digital methods when undertaking cross-national projects.

By considering the health and medical periodical's textual content alongside factors such as price, physical format, readership, and editorship, the contributors to this issue show how we are able to view these periodicals as dynamic, multi-vocal, multi-purpose publications—crucial not only to the personal career development of medical professionals but also to the cultivation of medical knowledge among the public. As many of the contributors here demonstrate, medical periodicals were not the preserve of doctors and nurses, but were also read by the general public; thus, the study of medical periodicals shows itself to be relevant to the study of nineteenth-century periodical culture as a whole.

Disclosure Statement

No potential conflict of interest was reported by the authors.

Funding

The Oxford workshop was funded by the John Fell Oxford University Press (OUP) Research Fund and co-organised by the Constructing Scientific Communities: Citizen Science in the 19th and 21st Centuries project, funded by the Arts and Humanities Research Council, Grant number AH/L007010/1 (https://conscicom.org/), and Diseases of Modern Life: Nineteenth-Century Perspectives, funded by the European Research Council under the Seventh Framework Programme, Grant number 340121 (https://diseasesofmodernlife.org/).

Notes

1. Bynum and Wilson note an acceleration in the growth of new titles in the last two decades of the century. Bynum and Wilson, "Periodical Knowledge," 30.
2. *Ibid.*
3. W.F. Bynum, Stephen Lock and Roy Porter, "Introduction," 4.
4. Patton, "Not a Limitless Possession"; Furlong, "Health Advice in Popular Periodicals."
5. Pladek, "A Variety of Tastes," 576; Brown "Bats, Rats and Barristers," 184.
6. Berkowitz, *Charles Bell and the Anatomy of Reform*, 76–102.

7. Referring to the *Lancet's* firebrand founding editor, Thomas Wakley, Bynum, Lock and Porter observed that 'by historical sleight of hand, the history of British medical journalism becomes dissolved into the career of Thomas Wakley'. Bynum, Lock and Porter, "Introduction," 2. Today the *Lancet* continues to wield influence, and has the second highest impact factor of any medical journal in the world; "The Lancet," accessed 6 September 2016, http://www.thelancet.com/lancet/about.

8. Hobbs, "The Deleterious Dominance of *The Times*," 491.

9. Milligan, "Illusionary Order," 544.

10. Toon, Timmermann and Worboys, "Text-Mining and the History of Medicine."

Bibliography

Berkowitz, Carin. *Charles Bell and the Anatomy of Reform*. Chicago: University of Chicago Press, 2016.

Brown, Michael. "'Bats, Rats and Barristers': *The Lancet*, Libel and the Radical Stylistics of Early Nineteenth-Century English Medicine." *Social History* 39 (2014): 189–209.

Bynum, W.F, Stephen Lock, and Roy Porter. "Introduction." In *Medical Journals and Medical Knowledge: Historical Essays*, edited by W. F. Bynum, Stephen Lock, and Roy Porter, 1–5. London: Routledge, 1992.

Bynum, W.F, and Janice Wilson. "Periodical Knowledge: Medical Journals and Their Editors in Nineteenth-Century Britain." In *Medical Journals and Medical Knowledge: Historical Essays*, edited by W. F. Bynum, Stephen Lock, and Roy Porter, 29–48. London: Routledge, 1992.

Furlong, Claire. "Health Advice in Popular Periodicals: Reynold's Miscellany, the Family Herald, and Their Correspondents." *Victorian Periodicals Review* 49, no. 1 (2016): 28–48.

Hitchcock, Tim. "Academic History Writing and its Disconnects." *Journal of Digital Humanities* 1, no. 1 (2011). Accessed September 7, 2016. http://journalofdigitalhumanities.org/1-1/academic-history-writing-and-its-disconnects-by-tim-hitchcock/.

Hobbs, Andrew. "The Deleterious Dominance of *The Times* in Nineteenth-Century Scholarship." *Journal of Victorian Culture* 18, no. 4 (2013): 472–496.

Milligan, Ian. "Illusionary Order: Online Databases, Optical Character Recognition, and Canadian History, 1997-2010." *The Canadian Historical Review* 94, no. 4 (2013): 540–569.

Patton, Cynthia Ellen. "'Not a Limitless Possession' Health Advice and Reader's Agency in The Girls' Own Paper, 1880-1890." *Victorian Periodicals Review* 45, no. 2 (2012): 111–133.

Pladek, Brittany. "'A Variety of Tastes': The Lancet in the Early-Nineteenth-Century Periodical Press." *Bulletin of the History of Medicine* 85, no. 4 (2011): 560–586.

Toon, Elizabeth, Carsten Timmermann, and Michael Worboys. "Text-Mining and the History of Medicine: Big Data, Big Questions?" *Medical History* 60, no. 2 (2016): 294–296.

THE 'MEDICAL-WOMEN QUESTION' AND THE MULTIVOCALITY OF THE VICTORIAN MEDICAL PRESS, 1869–1900

Alison Moulds ⓘ

From the late 1860s to 1900s, the British medical press was preoccupied by debates about the suitability and propriety of women studying and practising medicine. Rather than presenting a unitary or fixed opinion on the 'medical-women question', however, the journals illustrate divisions and dissent. Editorial opinions on the matter—expressed in leading articles and news coverage—were often strident, but were also revised and even reversed in later issues. Discussions of the medical-women movement also featured elsewhere in the journals, in transcripts of debates among professional bodies and correspondence pages. This enabled a range of individuals—professionals and laypeople, men and women, supporters and detractors—to participate in the conversation. The journals engaged with a spectrum of opinions, which reveal much about professional anxieties and attitudes towards women during this period. The medical press did not simply reflect contemporary values, however. Rather its multivalent form actively engendered debates about women in medicine.

'The medical-women question is perennial. It knows no limits; we encounter it at every turn.'[1]

In this editorial, published in 1877, the *Lancet* suggested that debates regarding the suitability and propriety of women studying and practising medicine had become pervasive. Readers would have been well aware of the subject's ubiquity, given that it appeared with remarkable frequency in the pages of the journal itself. Indeed, from the 1860s to well into the twentieth century, the 'medical-women question' received extensive coverage across the professional press.

This article examines how the medical-women movement was constructed and contested across a range of general medical journals. It explores long-running and widely-read titles such as the *Lancet* (1823-), *British Medical Journal* (*BMJ*, 1857-), and *Medical Press and Circular* (*MPC*, 1867–1961), as well as shorter-lived periodicals such as the *Medical Times and Gazette* (*MTG*, 1852–85) and the lesser-known *Medical Mirror* (*MM*, 1864–70). These journals represented various professional interests and were in direct competition in the periodical marketplace.

The *Lancet,* founded by surgeon Thomas Wakley in 1823, gained notoriety as a bold agitator for medical reform, though its zealous tone tempered after the early decades. Wakley died in 1862, but the journal remained in the family's hands until 1909. Until the

1870s, it enjoyed the largest circulation of any medical periodical.[2] In 1827, several metropolitan luminaries formed the *London Medical Gazette* in direct opposition to the *Lancet*. In 1852, it amalgamated with the *Medical Times* (established 1839) to form the *MTG*. Over its three decades in publication, the combined journal remained a leading competitor to Wakley's journal.[3] The *BMJ*, the mouthpiece of the British Medical Association, eventually surpassed the *Lancet* in popularity. It was a continuation of the *Provincial Medical and Surgical Journal* (1840–52) and the *Association Medical Journal* (1853–6). Its original aim was to represent the interests of provincial practitioners, but it increasingly spoke for the wider profession and soon moved its editorial operations to London. Between 1867–9 and 1870–98, it was edited by surgeon Ernest Hart. Like Wakley, Hart was something of a campaigning journalist.[4] Another journal which gradually became more metropolitan in character was the *MPC*. It started in Ireland as the *Dublin Medical Press* (1839). In 1866, this journal purchased (and combined with) the *Medical Circular* (established 1852). From 1868 onwards, it was published in London, though between 1860–1901 it was edited by Archibald Jacob, a prominent ophthalmologist in Dublin.[5]

Much less is known about the *MM*, a London-based journal which proudly proclaimed itself an 'independent organ'. It was edited by metropolitan physician William Abbotts Smith and later Alexander Thorburn Macgowan, who had served as Staff-Surgeon in the 52nd Oxfordshire Light Infantry. The journal's last editor—who oversaw production between September 1869 and December 1870—was anonymous and has not been identified.

These disparate titles varied in their political leanings, editorial strategies, and tone. Nevertheless, they were united by their engagement with the medical-women question. Their response to the issue cannot neatly be tied to their individual editors or character. As this article shows, the journals represented a spectrum of opinions and a multiplicity of voices. During the period from 1869 to 1900, all these titles were printed weekly, except for the *MM*, which appeared monthly. This article primarily draws on high-frequency journals because they could respond more quickly to developments in the medical-women movement.

During the second half of the nineteenth century, women made considerable inroads into the medical profession in Britain and its Empire. In 1865, there were just two women on the Medical Register in Britain—Elizabeth Blackwell and Elizabeth Garrett (later Garrett Anderson)—both of whom entered through loopholes, which were subsequently closed to prevent other women following suit.[6] In 1869–70, Sophia Jex-Blake and several female peers fought to pursue a medical education at the University of Edinburgh. If successful, they would have become the first women to take medical degrees from a British university. It was at this time that the professional press began treating the woman-doctor question with real immediacy and urgency. Although ultimately barred from graduating, these early pioneers paved the way for reform. In 1876, the Enabling Act officially sanctioned (though did not compel) medical schools to examine women and a year later the King and Queen's College of Physicians of Ireland became the first of the UK's nineteen licensing bodies to open its examinations to women. Gradually, other institutions accepted women, and by 1892 there were 135 female practitioners on the Register.[7]

Rather than treating the medical-women movement as a narrative of progress, this article explores the way in which the subject remained contentious throughout the period. Since the movement advanced unevenly, the journals found it difficult to establish a fixed and comprehensive response to the medical-women question. In the 1850s–60s, the debate centred on women's suitability for studying medicine, but it increasingly broached wider questions about where women might practise. During the 1880s–90s, attention shifted to their (un)suitability for Government appointments or work in the British Empire, for instance. At the *fin de siècle*, debates focused on whether they should be admitted to professional organisations such as the British Medical Association and the Royal Colleges. Across the period, the journals grappled with different implications of the medical-women movement.

Pioneering medical women have long been the subject of biographical study, but only in recent decades has the wider movement attracted significant scholarly attention. Historians have examined the experiences of early cohorts of female medical students and practitioners,[8] while literary critics have studied the representation of medical women in fiction.[9] Research has begun to consider how the medical-women question was mediated through periodicals. Thomas Neville Bonner's comparative study of women's medical education across European and North American contexts looks at how the popular and medical press responded to developments.[10] Laura Kelly examines coverage in the British and Irish popular and professional press, arguing that contemporary hostilities towards medical women illustrate anxieties about femininity and the continued investment in women's roles as wives and mothers.[11] Analysing the *Lancet*'s treatment of the issue between the 1860s–80s, Claire Brock contends that medical men were preoccupied by the question, but that they were neither 'coherent [n]or unified in [their] objections'. She argues that these inconsistencies reveal much about the profession's anxieties regarding its own status during this period.[12] For these scholars, the medical press' mixed coverage demonstrates how ideas about the medical profession and womanhood were under revision.

The journals reflected anxieties about whether the demands of medicine and femininity could be reconciled. However, they did not simply react to developments in the medical-women movement but instead actively set the terms of the debate. Building on previous research, this article interrogates what the medical journals' handling of the woman-doctor question suggests about their form and content and their community of readers. It draws on scholarship about nineteenth-century periodical culture. Critics have discussed the role journals played in shaping contemporary ideologies. For example, in their analysis of gender and the periodical press, Hilary Fraser, Stephanie Green, and Judith Johnston suggest that the genre's 'ephemeral character' rendered it 'an apt mediating agency for the presentation of ideas that were constantly undergoing revision and reformulation'.[13] Research has also demonstrated the multivocal nature of nineteenth-century journals, including the medical press.[14] Laurel Brake, Bill Bell, and David Finkelstein discuss how—through attempts to attribute articles to specific authors—'the formerly monovocal periodical text' has been revealed as 'a site for competing voices, contending within and even, at times, reorienting the very textual spaces they occupy'.[15]

This article traces coverage of the medical-women movement across the different journals and within individual titles. It engages with a cross-section of content and a range of voices, to understand how they interacted with one another. The article begins by looking at leading articles and news columns, where an editorial voice was either implicit or explicit. It then considers how the issue appeared in transcripts of debates at professional bodies and in correspondence columns. Finally, the article interrogates the role of female voices in the medical press. Ultimately, it considers how the journals—their constituent parts and the various voices contained within them—framed and re-framed the medical-women question. By suggesting that each development in the movement raised fundamentally new questions about women's participation in medicine, the journals ensured that the question remained fraught until the century's close.

Leading articles and news columns

Leading articles and news columns seemed to function as a journal's editorial mouthpiece.[16] Since they usually appeared anonymously, with leaders conventionally positioned beneath the journal's title, their commentary on current affairs seemed to represent editorial opinion or policy. Leading articles were usually overtly polemical, and variously adopted liberal, moderate, or conservative standpoints. While news stories were regularly printed without direct editorial intervention, they often contained asides which made their opinion on the story implicit or explicit.

At times, journals self-consciously identified themselves as either sympathetic or hostile towards the movement. In 1869, the *MM* indicated its tentative support for medical women. It positioned itself in direct opposition to some of its contemporaries, deriding the *MTG* for its 'pseudo-scientific dogmas' about women's 'physical and mental capacity' and the *BMJ* for its 'medieval notions concerning women'.[17] This demonstrates how journals were keenly aware of the content published by their rivals and how they sought to create an identity which would distinguish them in the crowded periodical market.

As the *MM* suggests, in the early years of the movement the *BMJ* presented itself as openly opposed to the prospect of women in medicine. In 1870, it featured a particularly histrionic editorial, which branded the 'lady-doctor' a 'traitress to her sex'. The article insisted that a civilised society should see women dependent on men, rather than following their own 'eccentric longing[s] for the will-o'-the-wisp pleasures of independence'.[18] A month later, another editorial suggested that the medical-women movement was a sign of 'retrograde civilisation'. It listed seven reasons why female practitioners were unnecessary or undesirable, including the fact that the medical profession was 'already well supplied as to numbers'.[19]

Editorial opinions were not always straightforward. In a pair of leading articles published in February 1870, the *MPC* equivocated over the question of women's suitability for medicine. It suggested that, in the spirit of 'toleration', women should be allowed to pursue a medical education, but it doubted whether they would succeed in practice.[20] These articles drew on ideas of justice and fair play, which were seen as important for a profession divesting itself of its old associations with trade and establishing its respectability.[21] In *Book on The Physician Himself* (1882), a popular advice manual for medical men originally published in the US, Daniel Webster Cathell emphasised that '[t]oleration of a difference of opinion is a lofty virtue'.[22]

Across the medical journals, editorial opinions showed vacillations, revisions and retrenchments. Rather than establishing a fixed standpoint, leaders often demonstrated indecision and inconsistency. Over time, this could be attributed to changes in editorship or the fact that different writers may have been supplying the copy. In 1866, the *MM* had exhibited reservations about women practising medicine, arguing that, 'while cultivating their minds', women should not 'neglect a department of usefulness for which Nature has peculiarly fitted them'; a reference to reproduction and childrearing.[23] Much of its positive coverage of the movement followed the departure of Macgowan as editor. The September 1869 issue signalled that he had retired and sold the copyright.[24] The new (anonymous) editor implicitly adopted a more liberal agenda, sympathetic towards medical women. Without knowing his identity, it is difficult to determine the reasons for his support. Since the *MM* ceased publication in 1870, one cannot know whether this editorial opinion would have been sustained. Perhaps it contributed to the journal's decline.

The *BMJ*'s cluster of articles antagonistic towards the movement appeared under the editorship of Jonathan Hutchinson, an eminent surgeon. He conducted the journal between late 1869 and the summer of 1870, during the short-lived absence of Hart. Peter Bartrip's history of the *BMJ* describes how Hutchinson staunchly opposed the medical women, whereas attitudes tempered under Hart, a friend of Garrett Anderson.[25] Despite this shift in opinion, readers may have considered the early editorials as the *BMJ*'s definitive stance on the medical-women question.

Even journals which remained under more continuous editorship—such as the *Lancet*—also reversed their opinions, sometimes in a matter of several weeks. As Brock illustrates, there were 'fluctuations and inconsistencies' in its editorial opinion.[26] In March 1870, the journal appeared to concede that the diseases of women and children would be 'the most appropriate field' for female practitioners.[27] This was the specialty that aspiring medical women usually claimed as their especial province, arguing that modest or delicate women might be reluctant to receive male attendance. However, two months later the journal effectively backtracked, suggesting that there would be no appetite for female practitioners among female patients. In a particularly vituperative leading article, it claimed that 'women hate one another, often at first sight, with a rancour of which men can form only a faint conception'.[28]

In a later editorial, the *Lancet* denied its opposition to women entering the profession stemmed from pettiness or self-protectionism. In 1875, amidst legislative change, it stated that it was not afraid of competition 'in the form of girl-graduates'. Given that the *Lancet* had a reputation for a radical and reformist agenda, it is perhaps unsurprising that it wished to disassociate itself from charges of exclusivity. Instead, it portentously warned that women in medicine would 'mark a new era in social and political history'.[29] The article deferred taking a position by re-framing the question of women's entry to the Medical Register as one with far-reaching ramifications.

Journals also distinguished between different aspects of the medical-women question, thus assuaging suspicions that they might be vacillating. In 1884, when the *Lancet* addressed the issue of female practitioners in India, it suggested that,

Nothing that has ever been urged in these columns against the pretensions of women to engage in the study and practice of medicine can be held to apply to the case of those countries in which women are as a sex secluded or so far kept apart that [medical] men may not minister to their needs.[30]

Medical women were often seen as making necessary or worthwhile contributions to colonial healthcare, particularly following the inauguration of the National Association for Supplying Female Medical Aid to the Women of India in 1885. This scheme employed female practitioners to work among the native women of India, who—it was widely held—were unable to receive male medical attendance due to their observance of purdah or zenana (practices of veiling or seclusion).

In general, medical journals tempered their stance towards medical women in the closing decades of the century. However, it should not be presumed that they became uniformly more tolerant. Certain aspects of the medical-women question continued to vex some journals, while others were apparently untroubled. In 1883, several of the journals' news columns reported on the Government's appointment of a female practitioner (Edith Shove) to attend the Post Office's female staff. The *Lancet* was aghast; in two separate items in its 'Annotations' column it questioned the propriety of the appointment, suggesting it might not be 'agreeable' to the patients' wishes. It thereby subverted medical women's claims about patient preference.[31] The *BMJ*, however—once an outspoken critic of the medical-women movement—reported on the same news without comment.[32] Less than a decade later it was similarly unperturbed by a decidedly more contentious issue: the prospect of women doctors taking up appointments relating to a mixed-sex patient constituency.[33] This indicates the journal's increasingly progressive stance towards medical women under Hart's editorship.

It is apparent that medical journals not only held divergent opinions to one another, but also contained internal inconsistencies. Even in features traditionally associated with editorial opinion and policy—such as leading articles and news columns—the medical press emerges as a fragmented genre. Historical and literary researchers must bear in mind that one editorial does not necessarily represent that journal's opinion. Indeed, decontextualising individual articles risks oversimplifying the dynamics of the press, where the treatment of medical women was remarkably fluid. This impression was reinforced by the fact that the journals contained many other voices (separate from the editor's own) commenting on the issue.

Transcripts of debates

One regular feature of the medical press that was inherently and explicitly multivocal was the transcripts of debates that took place among medical societies and professional bodies. These were published by the *Lancet* and *BMJ* in a seemingly verbatim format, taking the form of reported (apparently unexpurgated) speech, attributed to named persons. While there is a sense that the content has been mediated by a secretary or reporter—the third-person used instead of personal pronouns, for instance—these features grant access to the voices of a range of individuals. Throughout this period, professional bodies debated various aspects of the medical-women question. The transcripts illustrate the multiplicity and diversity of opinions that were aired, both between different organisations and within them.

In 1875, the General Medical Council (GMC) was tasked by the Government to produce a report on the prospect of medical women's registration, ahead of legislation that resulted in the Enabling Act. The GMC debated the issue in depth, with members touching on issues ranging from the propriety of co-education to women's physical and mental capability for practice, and whether there was sufficient appetite for their services. In a lengthy speech, Edinburgh-based surgeon Andrew Wood argued that 'women are not adapted to the medical profession and the medical profession is not adapted to women'. His contention that medicine and femininity were essentially incompatible resurfaced in myriad guises over the decades. Nevertheless, despite vocal opposition, the GMC finally agreed that its report should include the statement that it was 'not prepared to say that women ought to be excluded from the profession'.[34]

In the 1890s, the British Medical Association (BMA), the Royal College of Physicians of London (RCP), and the Royal College of Surgeons of England (RCS) all debated whether to admit women as members of their organisations. At an Extraordinary General Meeting (EGM) in 1892, the BMA voted in favour, while in 1895 both Royal Colleges voted against. These debates demonstrate the variety of arguments put forward against medical women at a relatively late stage in the movement, once a considerable number had already qualified, registered, and set up in practice.

The transcripts attest that some medical men believed women doctors had already proven themselves. During the BMA's EGM, Surrey-based GP John Henry Galton contended that '[t]he question against the general admission of women to the profession no longer existed' and 'all that remained was that they should be admitted freely'.[35] However, others were unconvinced by women's fitness for medical practice and professional membership. At the BMA, Dr Samuel Haughton from the University of Dublin claimed that the presence of women would 'diminish [the Association's] opportunities of discussing questions in that thorough and complete manner that science required'.[36] Anxieties about exchanging ideas in a mixed-sex environment recall fears about co-educational medical classes, the supposed impropriety of women and men learning anatomy alongside one another. Meanwhile, at the RCP debate, London-based physician Dr Charles John Hare suggested that women 'had no capacity for creating knowledge or advancing it'.[37] It is apparent that, by the 1890s, some regarded the medical-women question as already answered, while others saw these debates as an opportunity to revisit wider questions about women's fitness to participate in the profession.

Exceptionally and rather ironically, a medical woman was able to take part in the BMA debate. In 1874, the Association had accepted Garrett Anderson as a member through an 'oversight' before it officially vetoed the admission of further women four years later.[38] When the issue resurfaced in 1892, Garrett Anderson utilised her unique platform to argue for the rights of her female colleagues. She insisted that women's exclusion prevented them from cultivating 'any feeling of solidarity with other members of the profession', while also hampering them from extending their medical knowledge.[39] At a second EGM on the issue, Nelson Hardy (a Dulwich-based surgeon) praised Garrett Anderson, describing how she had conferred 'honour' on the BMA and the profession.[40] Both effectively suggested that women's involvement in the Association was in the profession's best interests.

By publishing transcripts, the medical press enabled those who were not present at the meetings to keep informed. Yet the journals were not simply vehicles for disseminating this material. Coverage of the debates spilled over into other sections, allowing different commentators to intercede with their views. Editorial columns engaged with the debates in detail. Reflecting on the Royal College debates, the *Lancet* noted that it was pleased the petitions were being discussed, since this indicated 'that the women are to have fair play'.[41] Following the debates, the *MPC* criticised arguments put forward against the women, which it claimed were based on 'sordid commercial ground' (i.e. designed to prevent women from competing in a crowded medical marketplace).[42] Here, both journals promote ideals of tolerance and fairness.

In the correspondence pages, there was extensive discussion about the outcome of the debates. The *BMJ* received numerous letters disputing the legitimacy of the BMA's vote.[43] This led to a second EGM which ratified the earlier decision.[44] Correspondents also revisited specific claims put forward about medical women's work. For instance, during the RCP discussion, Sir Joseph Fayrer—who had enjoyed an illustrious career in India—suggested that 'too much had been made' of the idea native women preferred the attendance of their own sex. He claimed that 'there was no difficulty in the way of medical men entering the most jealously guarded harem'.[45] After printing these comments, the *Lancet* received correspondence both welcoming and challenging his contention, which it published between November 1895 and February 1896.[46]

Ultimately, the debate transcripts were not static content. Editors intervened to comment on the discussions and readers actively engaged with the material. Tracking this coverage reveals the way in which the journals' heterogeneous content—their editorials, transcripts, and correspondence pages—closely interacted with one another. Conversations about debates that had taken place among professional organisations traversed separate sections of the journal and spread across different issues. Thus, even after votes had been cast, the debates were extended and reenergised within the pages of the medical press.

Correspondence

Correspondence pages were frequently sites for lively debate. Many of the journals published letters that represented a spectrum of opinions. At times, they printed those which accorded with their current editorial position. In the same issue in which the *Lancet* published its leading article suggesting there was no appetite for female practitioners since '[w]omen hate one another', it featured a letter ostensibly from a lay-woman, speaking out against the medical-women movement. Writing under the feminised pseudonym 'Mater', the correspondent asserted that '[m]orally, women are not fitted to be doctors, because they cannot (even the best of them) hold their tongues'.[47] The authenticity of this letter is questionable: was 'Mater' the pen-name of an ordinary woman who wished to express her distaste for the notion of female practitioners, or was it adopted by a disgruntled medical man seeking to discredit the campaign for women doctors? Regardless, the *Lancet* may have included the letter in this issue precisely because it seemed to offer further 'evidence' that medical women were unnecessary or undesirable.

Correspondents were not simply passive consumers of the journals, readily absorbing and reflecting their ideologies. Often they directly challenged the views expressed and journals engaged with ideas antithetical to their own. For instance, two weeks after querying whether there was any appetite for medical women, the *Lancet* printed a list of petitions organised by Sarah Kingsley (wife of the novelist Henry Kingsley, and a staunch supporter of the medical-women cause) in *favour* of female medical education.[48]

The correspondence columns offered medical women and their supporters an opportunity to share information and express their views. The *MTG*, for instance, enabled Garrett to advertise scholarships available to women.[49] Female students and practitioners were also able to rebut claims made against them by previous correspondents. In the *Lancet*, Jex-Blake countered suggestions that women could simply take up poorly-remunerated midwifery cases rather than pursuing full medical careers.[50] Later, Marion Ritchie (Honorary Secretary of Clapham Maternity Hospital and St John's Maternity, Battersea) refuted accusations that women were undercutting their male colleagues by offering midwifery services for low fees.[51] It is significant that midwifery was a bone of contention for it had traditionally been the preserve of women until the rise of the 'man-midwife' in the eighteenth century.[52]

Readers were not merely reactive to previously published content but played a vital role in generating and shaping debates. In 1869, the *MPC* ran correspondence on the medical-women question for some weeks, before wading in and issuing its own edict through two leading articles. It noted that it had already

> freely thrown open [its] columns to the advocates on both sides of the question [...] conceiving that, wherever the truth of the subject may lie, discussion, open and unfettered, is the one and only manner of reaching it.[53]

It is worth considering why the journal printed such an extensive range of correspondence before intervening. Perhaps—as it claimed—it wished to cultivate a sense of openness, or possibly it wanted to gauge readers' responses to the issue before formulating its own. The journal appeared to privilege its readers' voices by giving them the opportunity to set out their views first. The *MPC* did not use its leading articles to close down the debate and continued to print letters on the subject for several months.

What is significant about this run of correspondence in the *MPC* is the variety of voices featured. As well as printing letters from medical men both for and against the movement, the journal included two pieces of correspondence from a laywoman named Eliza Arnold (who insisted delicate women would prefer female attendance) and one from the widow of a Welsh country doctor, who queried whether she would be able to follow in her husband's footsteps.[54] Across the journals, a wide range of individuals— male and female, young and old, professionals and laypeople—participated in debates about the medical-women movement through the correspondence pages. If deemed authentic, then the contributions of women such as 'Mater' and Arnold offer a glimpse of patients' perspectives, which rarely feature in the professional press.

It is worth considering how such a range of people came into contact with professional journals. Discussing the late Victorian periodical *Woman*, Lynne Warren emphasises the utility of correspondence columns for complicating the image of the 'implied reader' put forward by the magazine. However, she also cautions against assuming that readers who chose to correspond were 'representative' of the general readership.[55] In the medical press, it seems likely that some correspondents on the medical-women question were regular readers and subscribers, while others were energised by this single issue. It can be difficult to determine their interest, for while some correspondents identified themselves by their name, qualification, and place of work, others wrote under names hard to trace or adopted pseudonyms, perhaps designed to conceal their gender or any vested interests. While questions concerning the authorship of letters cannot always be resolved, it is nevertheless apparent that the correspondence columns functioned as a richly multivalent space.

Warren also highlights the way in which *Woman*'s letters pages were 'highly self-referential [...] assuming an awareness of the various threads of discourse running throughout them'.[56] Editorial responses to readers' correspondence referred to other sections of the magazine, and readers commented on previously published material. The correspondence columns in the medical press worked in a similar way, fostering discussions that traversed different sections of the issue and that reached beyond the individual edition, as noted in the discussion of debate transcripts.

Editors selected, arranged, and potentially even modified the letters that appeared on the printed page to engender and regulate debate. They often encouraged back-and-forth letter-writing between correspondents. At times, there was direct editorial intervention in these exchanges. The *Lancet* featured correspondence from Ritchie and her detractors about midwifery fees across several issues. After printing a second letter from Ritchie, it intervened with the comment: 'This correspondence must now cease'.[57] The journal allowed Ritchie to engage in debate but also controlled her participation. This does not necessarily indicate suppression of the female voice, for the admonition was seemingly also directed towards her critics. Moreover, it was a standard line used to curtail ongoing debates between practitioners that might otherwise become too tedious or confrontational.[58]

The female voice

The voices that featured in the medical press were typically gendered. The transcripts show that, during the 1875 GMC debates on the registration of female practitioners, some male commentators suggested that they were unable to speak on behalf of women, while many claimed to be citing the opinions of women they knew. As demonstrated, journals occasionally contained correspondence from women, some of whom were self-conscious about their participation in a traditionally male textual space. For instance, 'Mater' began her letter by suggesting that she had 'misgiving as to a lady correspondent being admissible in [the journal's] pages'. However, she also used her status as a respectable woman to lend authority to her argument. In denying that there was any appetite among women for female practitioners, she claimed to speak for 'the wives and mothers of England'.[59] Writing from an opposing viewpoint, Arnold also implied that her gender conferred authority. She dismissed remarks made by a previous male correspondent, suggesting that 'the gentleman has very little knowledge of the wants and wishes of so large a class as the unmarried women of this country now constitutes'.[60] Women studying or practising medicine could assert their professional credentials to validate their participation in debates. This was not necessarily a mark of insecurity, for male correspondents regularly listed their qualifications or appointments.

Women's voices did not appear solely in the context of the correspondence pages or (more rarely) the debate transcripts. Towards the end of the century, the medical press included clinical contributions from women. For instance, the *British Gynaecological Journal* printed studies from Mary Scharlieb and Mary Dixon in the 1890s, several years before women were admitted to its Society in 1901.[61] The way in which women were able to publish their clinical reports and observations (alongside those of their male counterparts) suggests that they were valued not simply for their interactions with female patients but for their contributions to medical knowledge as well.

Historians have emphasised that women's engagement with the medical press was infrequent.[62] Anne Digby suggests that they preferred to contribute to the popular press, perhaps convinced they would find a more sympathetic audience there.[63] However, the inclusion of their voices in the medical journals remains significant given the opposition they faced in their attempts to enter other professional enclaves.

In order to examine how medical women constructed their own professional identities in this period, it is necessary to adopt a multi-source approach. For example, Vanessa Heggie uses (auto)biographies and archival material from medical institutions, as well as journal cuttings, to explore how the first tranche of female doctors portrayed themselves. Through this 'patchwork of sources', Heggie suggests that 'what emerges is a quite distinctive professional voice, an unapologetic self-identity as intelligent and ambitious'.[64] It is likely that this comes across more markedly in women doctors' private papers and their records from working in female-led institutions. These documents gave women space to express themselves without fear of criticism or rebuke. Nevertheless, print was an important medium for aspiring medical women to advance their views. Jex-Blake's polemical essay 'Medicine as a Profession for Women' (1869) and Margaret Todd's three-volume novel *Mona Maclean, Medical Student* (1892) demonstrate women's confident engagement with other forms of writing.

Examples of medical women's assertiveness can be found in the medical press, though this is only occasional, and their voices were frequently mediated or undermined by interventions from editors and other (usually male) readers. There is evidence that gender bias persists in the twenty-first-century professional press. In recent decades, researchers have shown that medical women continue to be relatively underrepresented in medical journals both as authors of original research articles and on editorial boards.[65]

Conclusion

Victorian medical journals have been viewed as instruments for professionalisation.[66] In cultivating a professional identity, however, they had to contend with provocative new developments—such as the medical-women movement—which threatened to divide opinion among practitioners. Tracing coverage of the medical-women movement belies any preconceptions of homogeneity across the professional press. It illustrates not only that journals held divergent views from one another but that there was dissent and discord within individual titles. Some journals initially positioned themselves as broadly sympathetic or hostile to the movement. However, coverage was generally mixed and inconsistent, particularly in many of the long-running titles.

The ubiquity of these debates demonstrates that there was considerable anxiety about both the role of women and the status of medicine. This article has argued that medical journals did not simply respond or react to debates but actively engendered them. This does not mean that the medical-women movement was contentious purely because of how it was handled or mediated by the professional press. Evidently women's entry into the medical profession was a fraught process, involving legislative change and revisions to institutional policies. However, the medical press did not strive to promote feelings of consensus or propose a clear-cut resolution to the issue.

Medical journals engaged with, and actively encouraged, a range of conflicting opinions on the suitability or desirability of women in medicine. By refashioning the medical-women question—suggesting that each development in the movement raised fundamentally *new* questions—the journals risked seeming inconsistent, but they also fostered an impression that their coverage of the issue was fresh and novel. Coverage of the issue was often sensationalist in tone. While the *MM* promoted the medical-women movement in its final years, by positioning itself against other titles it nevertheless cultivated a sense of discord, which made for stimulating reading. The mixed coverage of medical women—which traversed different sections and different issues of the journals—was designed to engage readers. This was an important strategy for journals to attract and retain subscribers in a competitive periodical market.

One must be cautious about using this single issue as an example of how the journals functioned. Not all medico-social subjects attracted such extensive coverage across different sections of the press, nor did they arouse such strong and divergent opinions. Other issues—such as non-paying patients or the disruption caused by patients who called at inconvenient times—generated more consensus. Yet the way in which the woman-doctor debates unfolded offers a fascinating insight into how the medical press operated as a multivalent space.

Despite their mixed coverage, the journals did not collapse into incoherency. Leading articles were usually written in a polemical tone, with a confident authorial voice that belied any sense of uncertainty or vacillation. Thus, while discrepancies in editorial opinion undoubtedly emerged, readers were reassured that the journal had a coherent identity. Leading articles, debate transcripts, and correspondence pages were packaged as discernibly different content, allowing readers to navigate between the divergent views expressed therein. The journals presented themselves as vehicles for the dissemination of different opinions. The way in which they incorporated a broad spectrum of voices was partly an effort to demonstrate their investment in values such as toleration and fair play. Readers were entrusted to form their own opinions about women's capabilities and the demands of medical practice.

The way in which the medical press revisited the medical-women question from different angles across time was enabled by the seriality of the form. To some extent, the journal was an ephemeral product; individual issues were superseded by new ones, and titles might be short-lived. Despite this, readers were not necessarily expected to forget previous content, nor did new material simply replace old. Throughout the coverage of the medical-women question there were continuous 'threads of discourse'.[67] Editors, contributors, and correspondents reflected on discussions that had previously taken place or anticipated where they might go in future. Conversations about the medical-women question intersected different items in the issue and interwove through different editions. Thus, while the journals to some extent capitalised on divergences among their readers for the sake of lively copy, they also incorporated these readers within an ongoing debate or discourse. This served to maintain readers' interest and create a shared professional community.

Acknowledgment

This article is based on research carried out as part of my DPhil, under the supervision of Professor Sally Shuttleworth and Dr Samuel Alberti. I am indebted to both for their support and advice. Thank you also to my peer reviewers for their invaluable advice which helped to strengthen this article.

Funding

This work was supported by the Arts and Humanities Research Council [grant number AH/L007010/1] and [grant number 1470901].

Disclosure statement

No potential conflict of interest was reported by the author.

Notes

1. "Medical Women," 659.
2. See Brake and Demoor, *Dictionary of Nineteenth-Century Journalism*, 343–4.
3. Ibid., 375–6.
4. Ibid., 78–9.
5. Ibid., 182.
6. Elizabeth Blackwell registered under a special clause in the Medical Act (1858) which permitted those who had a foreign medical degree and were already practising to register. Elizabeth Garrett threatened legal action against the Society of Apothecaries if they refused to allow her to sit their examination after studying privately. The Society later stipulated that only those who had studied at recognised medical schools were eligible for examination.
7. "Extraordinary General Meeting," 262.

8. Kelly, *Irish Women in Medicine*; Crowther and Dupree, *Medical Lives*.

9. Swenson, *Medical Women and Victorian Fiction*.

10. Bonner, *To the Ends of the Earth*.

11. Kelly, *Irish Women in Medicine*, 30–1.

12. Brock, "The *Lancet* and the Campaign Against," 132.

13. Fraser et al., "Introduction," 3.

14. Peterson, "Medicine," 22–42.

15. Brake et al., "Introduction," 4–5.

16. Brake and Demoor, *Dictionary of Nineteenth-Century Journalism*, 352.

17. "Notes and Comments: Female Physicians," 173.

18. "Lady Surgeons," 338–9.

19. "The Admission of Ladies," 474–5.

20. "Lady Doctors" (16 Feb 1870), 127–8; "Lady Doctors" (23 Feb 1870), 146–7.

21. Digby, *Making a Medical Living*, 6.

22. Cathell, *The Physician Himself*, 73.

23. "The Rights of Women," 506.

24. *Medical Mirror* (1 Sep 1869), 113.

25. Bartrip, *Mirror of Medicine*, 172–3.

26. Brock, "The *Lancet* and the Campaign Against," 142.

27. "Notes, Short Comments, and Answers: Lady Doctors," 400.

28. "The Medical Education of Women," 673.

29. "Admission of Women," 213.

30. "Women Doctors for Women," 580.

31. "Lady Doctor for the Post-Office," 112; "The Appointment of Miss Shove," 468.

32. *BMJ* (17 Mar 1883), 523.

33. "Medical Women as Workhouse Doctors," 371.

34. "The General Council," 56.

35. "Extraordinary General Meeting," 262.

36. "British Medical Association," 481.

37. "RCP of London: Debate on the Petition," 1125.

38. Described in footnote in "The Constitution of the BMA," 67.

39. "Extraordinary General Meeting," 263.

40. "British Medical Association," 481–2.

41. "Women and the RCP of London," 1115.

42. "Notes on Current Topics," 532–3. For discussion of overcrowding, see Digby, *Evolution of British General Practice*, 23–4.

43. See "Correspondence: The Admission of Women," 383–4; "The Constitution and Annual Meetings of the BMA," 420–1.

44. "BMA: Admission of Women," 481–2.

45. "RCP of London: Debate on the Petition," 1125.

46. See McReddie, "Women and the Profession in India," 197; Dhingra, "Women and the Profession in India," 450.

47. "Mater," "A Lady on Lady Doctors," 680.

48. Kingsley, "Notes, Short Comments, and Answers," 757.

49. Garrett, "Medical Scholarships for Women," 298.

50. Jex-Blake, "Women as Practitioners of Midwifery," 63.
51. Ritchie, "Correspondence: The Admission of Women," 1537–8.
52. See Wilson, *The Making of Man-Midwifery*.
53. "Lady Doctors," 127.
54. Arnold, "Women Physicians," 525; Arnold, "Lady Doctors," 176; "A Lady on Lady Doctors," 199.
55. Warren, "Reading the Correspondence Columns," 122, 124.
56. Ibid., 127–8.
57. Ritchie, "Correspondence: The Admission of Women," 1668.
58. See "Correspondence: The Title of 'Doctor'," 1216.
59. "Mater," "A Lady on Lady Doctors," 680.
60. Arnold, "Women Physicians," 525.
61. Scharlieb, "Notes of Three Cases of Hysterectomy," 100–1; Dixon, "Disease of the Ovary, Colloid Degeneration," 398–411.
62. Kelly, *Irish Women in Medicine*, 127.
63. Digby, *Making a Medical Living*, 292; Digby, *Evolution of British General Practice*, 156.
64. Heggie, "Women Doctors and Lady Nurses," 270.
65. Filardo et al., "Trends and Comparison"; Amrein et al., "Women Underrepresented on Editorial Boards."
66. Peterson, "Medicine," 37–8.
67. Warren, "Reading the Correspondence Columns," 127–8.

Bibliography

"The Admission of Ladies to the Profession." *BMJ* 1 (7 May 1870): 474–5.

"Admission of Women to the Medical Profession." *Lancet* 106 (7 Aug 1875): 213.

Amrein, K., A. Langmann, A. Fahrleitner-Pammer, T. R. Pieber, and I. Zollner-Schwetz. "Women Underrepresented on Editorial Boards of 60 Major Medical Journals." *Gender Medicine* 8 (2011): 378–87. doi:10.1016/j.genm.2011.10.007

"The Appointment of Miss Shove, M.B., to the Post Office." *Lancet* 121 (17 Mar 1883): 468.

Arnold, Eliza. "Correspondence: Lady Doctors." *MPC* 9 (2 Mar 1870): 176.

Arnold, Eliza. "Correspondence: Women Physicians." *MPC* 8 (29 Dec 1869): 525.

Bartrip, Peter W. J. *Mirror of Medicine: The BMJ, 1840–1990*. Oxford: Oxford University Press, 1990.

BMJ 1 (17 Mar 1883): 523.

Bonner, Thomas Neville. *To the Ends of the Earth: Women's Search for Education in Medicine*. Cambridge, MA: Harvard University Press, 1992.

Brake, Laurel, Bill Bell, and David Finkelstein, eds. "Introduction." In *Nineteenth-Century Media and the Construction of Identities*, 1–7. Basingstoke, Hampshire: Palgrave, 2000.

Brake, Laurel, and Marysa Demoor. *Dictionary of Nineteenth-Century Journalism in Great Britain and Ireland*. Gent: Academia Press, 2009.

"British Medical Association: Admission of Women." *BMJ* 2 (27 Aug 1892): 481–2.

Brock, Claire. "The *Lancet* and the Campaign Against Women Doctors, 1860–1880." In *(Re)Creating Science in Nineteenth-Century Britain*, edited by Amanda Mordavsky Caleb, 130–45. Newcastle: Cambridge Scholars, 2007.

Cathell, D. W. *Book on the Physician Himself*. Philadelphia: F.A. Davis, 1890.

"The Constitution and Annual Meetings of the British Medical Association: The Admission of Women to the Association: A Constitutional Argument." *BMJ* 2 (20 Aug 1892): 420–1.

"The Constitution of the BMA." *Supplement to the BMJ* 1 (14 Mar 1953): 67–9.

"Correspondence: The Admission of Women to the Association." *BMJ* 2 (13 Aug 1892): 383–4.

"Correspondence: The Title of 'Doctor'." *Lancet* 145 (11 May 1895): 1215–6.

Crowther, M. Anne, and Marguerite W. Dupree. *Medical Lives in the Age of Surgical Revolution.* Cambridge: Cambridge University Press, 2007.

Dhingra, B. L. "Correspondence: Women and the Profession in India." *Lancet* 147 (15 Feb 1896): 450.

Digby, Anne. *Making a Medical Living: Doctors and Patients in the English Market for Medicine, 1720–1911.* Cambridge: Cambridge University Press, 1994.

Digby, Anne. *The Evolution of British General Practice 1850–1948.* Oxford: Oxford University Press, 1999.

Dixon, Mary. "The Fourth Hitherto Undescribed Disease of the Ovary, Colloid Degeneration." *British Gynaecological Journal* 15 (Nov 1899): 398–411.

"Extraordinary General Meeting." *BMJ* 2 (30 July 1892): 262–4.

Filardo, G., B. da Graca, D. M. Sass, B. D. Pollock, E. B. Smith, and M. A. Marie Martinez. "Trends and Comparison of Female First Authorship in High Impact Medical Journals: Observational Study (1994–2014)." *BMJ* 352 (2016). doi:10.1136/bmj.i847.

Fraser, Hilary, Stephanie Green, and Judith Johnston, eds. "Introduction." In *Gender and the Victorian Periodical*, 1–25. Cambridge: Cambridge University Press, 2003.

Garrett, Elizabeth. "Notes, Queries, and Replies: Medical Scholarships for Women." *MTG* 2 (4 Sep 1869): 298.

"The General Council of Medical Education and Registration: Session 1875." *Lancet* 106 (10 July 1875): 55–63.

Heggie, Vanessa. "Women Doctors and Lady Nurses: Class, Education, and the Professional Victorian Woman." *Bulletin of the History of Medicine* 89, no. 2 (Summer 2015): 267–92.

Jex-Blake, Sophia. "Correspondence: Women as Practitioners of Midwifery." *Lancet* 96 (9 July 1870): 63–4.

Kelly, Laura. *Irish Women in Medicine, c.1880s-1920s: Origins, Education and Careers.* Manchester: Manchester University Press, 2012.

Kingsley, S. M. K. "Notes, Short Comments, and Answers to Correspondents." *Lancet* 95 (21 May 1870): 757.

"A Lady Doctor for the Post-Office." *Lancet* 121 (20 Jan 1883): 112.

"Lady Doctors." *MPC* 9 (16 Feb 1870): 127–8.

"Lady Doctors." *MPC* 9 (23 Feb 1870): 146–7.

"A Lady on Lady Doctors." *MPC* 9 (9 Mar 1870): 199.

"Lady Surgeons." *BMJ* 1 (2 Apr 1870): 338–9.

"Mater." "Correspondence: A Lady on Lady Doctors." *Lancet* 95 (7 May 1870): 680.

McReddie, G. D. "Correspondence: Women and the Profession in India." *Lancet* 147 (18 Jan 1896): 197.

"The Medical Education of Women." *Lancet* 95 (7 May 1870): 672–3.

Medical Mirror 6 (1 Sep 1869): 113.

"Medical Women." *Lancet* 110 (3 Nov 1877): 659.

"Medical Women as Workhouse Doctors." *BMJ* 1 (17 Feb 1894): 371.

"Notes and Comments: Female Physicians." *Medical Mirror* 6 (1 Dec 1869): 173.

"Notes on Current Topics: Admission of Women to the Profession." *MPC* 111 (20 Nov 1895): 532–3.

"Notes, Short Comments, and Answers to Correspondents: Female Medical Students." *Lancet* 96 (3 Dec 1870): 805.

"Notes, Short Comments, and Answers to Correspondents: Lady Doctors." *Lancet* 95 (12 Mar 1870): 400.

Peterson, M. Jeanne. "Medicine." In *Victorian Periodicals and Victorian Society*, edited by J. Don Vann, and Rosemary Van Arsdel, 22–42. Toronto: University of Toronto Press, 1994.

"The Rights of Women." *Medical Mirror* 3 (Aug 1866): 506.

Ritchie, Marion. "Correspondence: The Admission of Women to the Royal Colleges of Physicians of London and Surgeons of England." *Lancet* 146 (14 Dec 1895): 1537–8.

Ritchie, Marion. "Correspondence: The Admission of Women to the Royal Colleges of Physicians of London and Surgeons of England." *Lancet* 146 (28 Dec 1895): 1668.

"Royal College of Physicians of London: Debate on the Petition for Admission of Women to the Examinations and Diplomas." *Lancet* 146 (2 Nov 1895): 1125–7.

Scharlieb, Mary. "Notes of Three Cases of Hysterectomy." *British Gynaecological Journal* 12 (May 1896): 100–1.

Swenson, Kristine. *Medical Women and Victorian Fiction*. Columbia: University of Missouri Press, 2005.

Warren, Lynne. "'Women in Conference': Reading the Correspondence Columns in *Woman* 1890–1910." In *Nineteenth-Century Media and the Construction of Identities*, edited by Laurel Brake, Bill Bell, and David Finkelstein, 122–34. Basingstoke: Palgrave, 2000.

Wilson, Adrian. *The Making of Man-Midwifery: Childbirth in England, 1660–1770*. Cambridge, MA: Harvard University Press, 1995.

"Women and the Royal College of Physicians of London." *Lancet* 146 (2 Nov 1895): 1115.

"Women Doctors for Women." *Lancet* 123 (29 Mar 1884): 580.

SHAPING DOCTORS AND SOCIETY
The Portuguese Medical Press (1880–1926)

Ana Carneiro, Teresa Salomé Mota and **Isabel Amaral**

This article is an exploratory approach to the study of the Portuguese medical press, between the 1880s and 1926, that is, from the last decades of the liberal monarchy (1820–1910) to the end of the First Republic (1910–1926). Around 130 medical journals were identified so far. They were divided in groups according to the place of publication, and a typology was established based on two combined criteria—contents and affiliation. The weekly journal A Medicina Contemporâ- nea will be used as a sample, mainly because it exemplifies in a single journal the dual purpose of the Portuguese medical press taken as whole. The establishment of the medical press coincided with the emergence of mass press and doctors' engagement in laboratory-based medicine, and constituted an apparatus with two aims in mind: shaping doctors not only technically and scien- tifically, but also ideologically with the aim of creating a market for their profession, building up a medical community, and a social and cultural elite; shaping society and improving the 'race' by taking care of the bodies and minds of the Portuguese, organizing public opinion through ideologi- cal indoctrination, and influencing political decision-making to make a republic regime viable.

Introduction

Medical journals are invaluable sources for historians of medicine and science. In this article the Portuguese medical press, between the last decades of the liberal monarchy (1820–1910) and the First Republic (1910–1926) will be approached as an apparatus and characterized as an object of historical enquiry. The impressive extent and range of the Por- tuguese medical journals in the period under consideration—so far 130 medical journals have been identified in various libraries and catalogues[1]—raise important questions regarding their typology, contents, literary styles, editors and their respective motives and intents, authors, readership and markets. No archival material associated with the pub- lication of most of these journals has been found so far, and consequently this investigation relies primarily on the consideration of the journals themselves, a variety of coeval printed sources, and secondary literature. Not to mention limitations of space, the number and variety of periodicals, as well as historiographical questions, methodological choices and the selection of analytical categories, necessarily impart an exploratory character to this article. In addition, the wide range of issues that can be addressed from the vantage point of the medical press constitute a vast research program that transcends these pages and calls for the cooperation of scholars sharing periodicals as their common inter- est, in order to move beyond the recognized fragmentation of the field of periodical studies.[2]

Especially when periodicals are in digital form as is nowadays common,[3] although not in the Portuguese case, scholars usually mine journals for materials relating to their fields of enquiry. But as Lathan and Sholes point out they are usually unable to say much about the periodical as a whole, as they tend to see periodicals as 'containers' of pieces of information.[4] Similarly, the study of individual periodicals does not put scholars in the position of saying much about the constellations of related journals published in a particular time and place, and their collective, cultural and political significance. And this is precisely what this article aims to do, first by studying the medical press as a polyvalent apparatus composed of various segments, having cultural and political meaning, and second, by analysing a periodical that reflects the characteristics present together, or in part, in the Portuguese medical press.

In the period under consideration, doctors' quest for work, proper wages and social respectability in Europe coincided with the development of an industrialized mass press,[5] with repercussions in Portugal. From the mid-nineteenth century, a range of factors converged to change the Portuguese general press: several entrepreneurs realized that popular 'neutral' and cheap mass press was a lucrative business abroad, and decided to create local newspapers; a distinction was made, however, between a straightforward journalistic style and a literary and scholarly kind of journalism.[6] It was in this atmosphere that the local medical press, which, however, seemed far from a lucrative enterprise, emerged and developed, often blending the 'factual' and 'rational' with opinion making and a persuasive style.

In effect, notwithstanding collaborations in newspapers[7] and the publication of textbooks, booklets, travelogues and novels, Portuguese doctors created this wide range of medical periodicals, many dealing with a variety of topics that transcended medicine. We argue in this article that in this, they had two aims in mind: to shape doctors and surgeons not only scientifically and technically, but also ideologically, in order to manufacture 'perfect' physicians, to build up a medical community and a social and cultural elite. Simultaneously, they aimed to fashion society through ideological indoctrination and education, in this way preparing the ground for their professional, social and political intervention, with the purpose of improving the nation's bodies and minds, that is, the 'race.'[8]

In addition to the analysis of the Portuguese medical press taken as a whole, special emphasis will be given in this article to the journal *A Medicina Contemporânea. Hebdomadario Portuguez de Sciencias Medicas* (*Contemporary Medicine. Weekly Journal of Portuguese Medical Sciences*, hereafter *MC*) for a variety of reasons. *MC* was one of the leading and emblematic Portuguese medical periodicals of its kind in the period under consideration, became to some extent a template for other medical periodicals, had an exceptionally long life (Figure 1), and was initially edited by a group of influential and politically engaged figures in Portuguese medicine, most operating in Lisbon. *MC* was a member of the Portuguese Association of the Medical Press (hereafter PAMP) and the Association Internationale de la Presse Médicale (International Association of the Medical Press, hereafter IAMP) created in 1903. The latter organization was formed as a response to medicine's growing media coverage, and the tensions between journalists writing on medical topics and doctors writing as journalists, especially for medical magazines and the general press.[9] *MC*, in addition, defined two styles of medical journalism—a populist brand and a refined and more 'aristocratic' style, the latter becoming a reference for the medical elite of the First Republic, known as the 'Generation of 1911.'[10] Above all, *MC*

MEDICAL PERIODICALS PUBLISHED
BETWEEN 1870 AND 1930

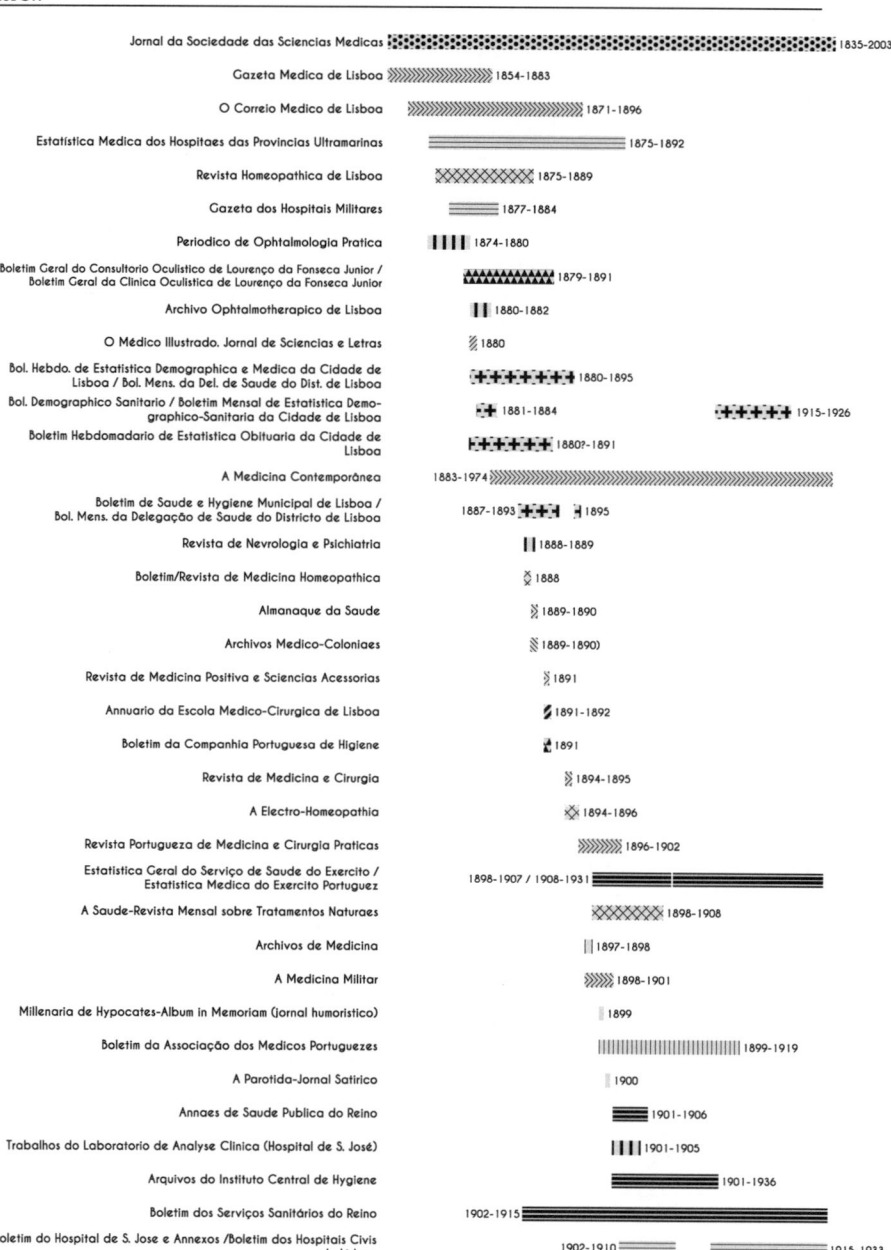

FIGURE 1

Portuguese medical journals launched between the 1870 and 1930, in Lisbon, Porto, Coimbra, provincial towns and cities, Portuguese colonies and abroad. In this article, only the journals published between the 1880s and 1926 are under consideration

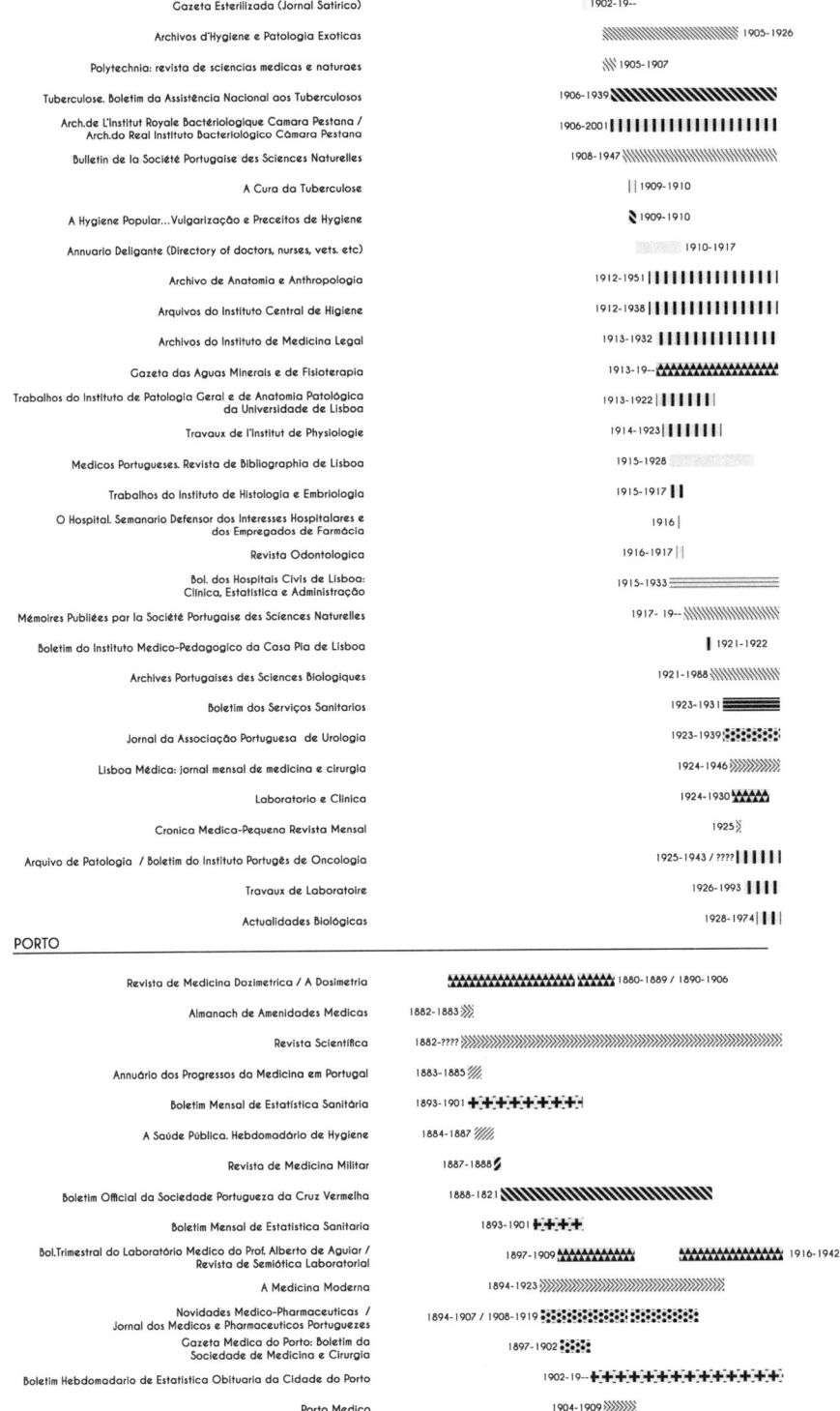

Gazeta Esterilizada (Jornal Satírico) — 1902-19--
Archivos d'Hygiene e Patologia Exoticas — 1905-1926
Polytechnia: revista de sciencias medicas e naturaes — 1905-1907
Tuberculose. Boletim da Assistência Nacional aos Tuberculosos — 1906-1939
Arch.de L'Institut Royale Bactériologique Câmara Pestana / Arch.do Real Instituto Bacteriológico Câmara Pestana — 1906-2001
Bulletin de la Société Portugaise des Sciences Naturelles — 1908-1947
A Cura da Tuberculose — 1909-1910
A Hygiene Popular...Vulgarização e Preceitos de Hygiene — 1909-1910
Annuario Deligante (Directory of doctors, nurses, vets. etc) — 1910-1917
Archivo de Anatomia e Anthropologia — 1912-1951
Arquivos do Instituto Central de Higiene — 1912-1938
Archivos do Instituto de Medicina Legal — 1913-1932
Gazeta das Aguas Minerais e de Fisioterapia — 1913-19--
Trabalhos do Instituto de Patologia Geral e de Anatomia Patológica da Universidade de Lisboa — 1913-1922
Travaux de l'Institut de Physiologie — 1914-1923
Medicos Portugueses. Revista de Bibliographia de Lisboa — 1915-1928
Trabalhos do Instituto de Histologia e Embriologia — 1915-1917
O Hospital. Semanario Defensor dos Interesses Hospitalares e dos Empregados de Farmácia — 1916
Revista Odontologica — 1916-1917
Bol. dos Hospitais Civis de Lisboa: Clínica, Estatística e Administração — 1915-1933
Mémoires Publiées par la Société Portugaise des Sciences Naturelles — 1917- 19--
Boletim do Instituto Medico-Pedagogico da Casa Pia de Lisboa — 1921-1922
Archives Portugaises des Sciences Biologiques — 1921-1988
Boletim dos Serviços Sanitarios — 1923-1931
Jornal da Associação Portuguesa de Urologia — 1923-1939
Lisboa Médica: jornal mensal de medicina e cirurgia — 1924-1946
Laboratorio e Clinica — 1924-1930
Cronica Medica-Pequena Revista Mensal — 1925
Arquivo de Patologia / Boletim do Instituto Portugês de Oncologia — 1925-1943 / ????
Travaux de Laboratoire — 1926-1993
Actualidades Biológicas — 1928-1974

PORTO

Revista de Medicina Dozimetrica / A Dosimetria — 1880-1889 / 1890-1906
Almanach de Amenidades Medicas — 1882-1883
Revista Scientifica — 1882-????
Annuário dos Progressos da Medicina em Portugal — 1883-1885
Boletim Mensal de Estatística Sanitária — 1893-1901
A Saúde Pública. Hebdomadário de Hygiene — 1884-1887
Revista de Medicina Militar — 1887-1888
Boletim Oficial da Sociedade Portugueza da Cruz Vermelha — 1888-1821
Boletim Mensal de Estatistica Sanitaria — 1893-1901
Bol.Trimestral do Laboratório Medico do Prof. Alberto de Aguiar / Revista de Semiótica Laboratorial — 1897-1909 / 1916-1942
A Medicina Moderna — 1894-1923
Novidades Medico-Pharmaceuticas / Jornal dos Medicos e Pharmaceuticos Portuguezes — 1894-1907 / 1908-1919
Gazeta Medica do Porto: Boletim da Sociedade de Medicina e Cirurgia — 1897-1902
Boletim Hebdomadario de Estatistica Obituaria da Cidade do Porto — 1902-19--
Porto Medico — 1904-1909

FIGURE 1
Continued

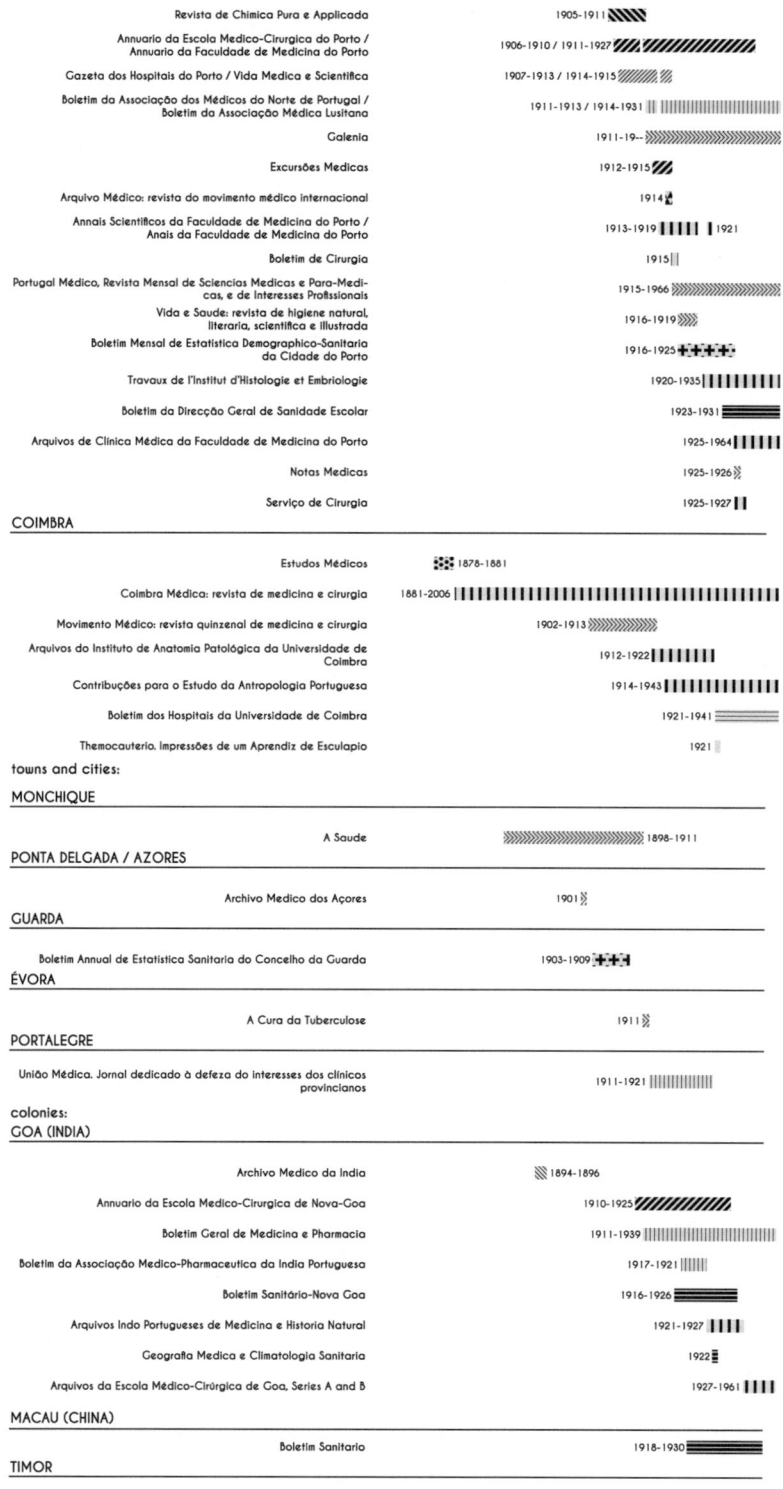

FIGURE 1
Continued

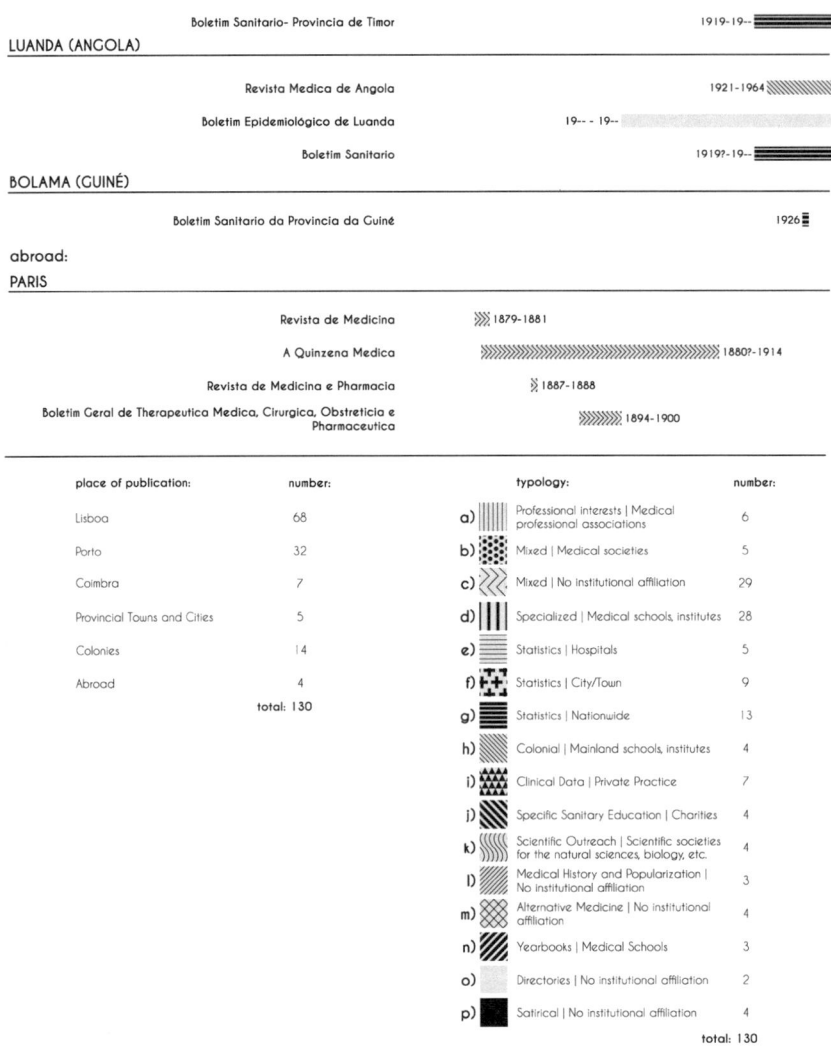

FIGURE 1
Continued

had a dual character and exemplified in a single journal the above-mentioned twofold aim of the Portuguese medical press: the presentation of medical articles *stricto sensu* targeted to a medical readership, and texts with great ideological and political content addressed to doctors and society in general. Thus, it will be used here as a sample and object of a more detailed albeit brief analysis in the latter aspect.

Although a significant part of the contents of Portuguese medical journals including *MC* could be classified as the 'popularization' of medicine and science—naturally bearing in mind the multiple debates around this concept, including in the 'peripheries'[11]—in the context of this study, 'propaganda' is undoubtedly more appropriate.[12] As argued elsewhere, not only was the latter a contemporary actors' term in the period under consideration,[13] which they were keen to distinguish from advertisement, but it better conveys their motivations, beliefs and clear intent of inculcating an ideology, as well as the strategies of persuasion put in place by Portuguese doctors in the medical press.

In effect, if in Portugal and elsewhere the laboratory became in this period the place where medical knowledge was built up and legitimized, we argue that the Portuguese medical press was no less relevant. It constituted a means of communication between doctors and this professional group and society, as well as an instrument to promote social, cultural and political change. It follows that when taken globally the Portuguese medical press was an apparatus, a 'propaganda machine' to 'manufacture consent'[14] around not only medical issues, but also the need for a new political regime, the republic. In this context, the ideology associated with the Portuguese intellectual movements that marked this period prepared the ground for action, notably the 'explosion' of medical journals. These promoted new legislation and regulations regarding education, medical education and training, public health, and medical practice; the launching of learned societies and professional medical associations, as well as the construction and organization of medical facilities in the three main cities (Lisbon, Porto and Coimbra), but most especially in Lisbon.[15]

Intellectual Movements and the Emergence of the Portuguese Medical Press

The emergence of the Portuguese medical press was a response to various challenges affecting society and was associated with intellectual movements, notably the 'Generation of 1870'[16] together with its sequels, the 'Defeated by Life' (Vencidos da Vida) (1887–1894), and the 'Generation of 1911.'[17] The former analysed the causes of the alleged decline of Portuguese society after the sixteenth century,[18] and was composed mainly of writers inclined to utopian socialism and republicanism, which crystallized respectively in the Socialist Party, in 1875, and the Republican Party, in 1876.

Subsequently, the country was marked by multiple political and economic crises: the 'scramble for Africa' (1881–1914); the partial bankruptcy, from 1891 to 1902; the regicide in 1908; the establishment of the First Republic, in 1910; and finally, the effects of the First World War. Thus, from the 1880s, the practitioners of what they termed 'learned medicine' ('medicina culta')—which, in this context, meant medicine legitimized by the laboratory as the place of objective scientific medical enquiry[19]—presented themselves, notably in the medical press, as agents of transformation and progress. Their ideas were informed by materialism, positivism and biological scientism, a social-political philosophy in which science was not only regarded as a substitute for religion,[20] but also as the driving force to achieve prosperity and social transformation.

In medical education, clinical practice and research, the laboratory emerged then as a source of scientific and professional authority. It became a key element in building up medical expertise founded on a body of abstract knowledge, science-based thinking and practices, all concurring to build up doctors' professional 'jurisdiction,'[21] socially legitimize their profession, and attain political influence, the medical press being instrumental in this respect. They saw themselves as especially prepared to counteract the degeneration of the 'race,' and ameliorate it in two fundamental ways: by taking care of the health and improving the bodies of the Portuguese, notably through public health, eugenics, and the creation of medical infrastructures; and by looking after their minds through education and propaganda to make a republican regime viable.[22]

By the early twentieth century, a new intellectual movement emerged, the 'Generation of 1911,' composed of doctors that built on the work of their predecessors and sided with the newly established republican regime. They were associated with the histo-physiology research school established in the Lisbon Medical-Surgical School (hereafter LMSS) by Marck Athias (1875–1946). He had been a disciple of Mathias Duval at the Faculty of Medicine of Paris,[23] revered the Spanish Nobel laureate Santiago Ramon y Cajal and admired German science and culture, rather than French, probably echoing the debates in France on the alleged superiority of German science and culture.[24] Athias and his disciples engaged in scientific propaganda, a term they themselves used, by writing for the daily press, delivering public lectures, publishing books and creating new medical and scientific journals in Lisbon. [25] Like their predecessors of the 1880s, they presented themselves as organizers of the scientific community and public opinion, becoming what Antonio Gramsci termed 'organic intellectuals,' seeking to produce 'hegemony,' that is, intellectual, moral, and ideological superiority.[26] Also like the former generation, through propaganda in the medical press and in newspapers they disseminated an ideology within the Portuguese medical community and spread it beyond its borders.[27]

Medical Journals, a Typology

Although the periodicals in the period under consideration fall into the categories of journal, magazine, newspaper, gazette, bulletin, yearbook, etc., with all of the problems classifications entail,[28] a distinct typology was established. Despite individual specifities many periodicals shared common features that were used to establish the groups and typology presented here (Figure 1), which, nevertheless, is bound to subsequent refinements, deriving from further research. Thus, with the available data, six groups of periodicals were formed according to the place of publication, and a typology was established based on two combined criteria, contents and affiliation, each type represented in a distinct pattern and a corresponding letter (Figure 1).

Amongst the 130 medical journals identified so far, between the 1880s and 1926, 107 were published in the three main Portuguese cities where medicine was taught: in the Faculty of Medicine of the University of Coimbra (hereafter FMUC), and at the LMSS and Porto Medical-Surgical School (PMSS), both created in 1836.[29] The latter were converted into Faculties of Medicine by the republican reform of education in 1911, which established the Universities of Lisbon and Porto. The distribution of the medical journals in time has two booming moments: one following the above mentioned 'Generation of 1870,' until the turn of the century, the whole period coinciding with the growth of republic movements; then, again, in the early years following the establishment of the First Republic.

In the spatial distribution of journals published in mainland Portugal, the colonies and abroad (Figure 1), Lisbon, the political capital then in the process of becoming also the scientific and intellectual capital and in this way hegemonic,[30] stands out with 68 medical journals, 24 being short-lived (that is, published for less than five years). It isfollowed by the second largest city, Porto, with 32 medical periodicals, 11 short-lived;

Coimbra, with the oldest Faculty of Medicine in the country, came third with seven journals, two short-lived. Five medical periodicals were published in mainland provincial cities; 14 in the colonies. Goa in India, where since 1842 a medical school established in Bambolim trained and supplied doctors to Portuguese India and the African colonies,[31] emerges as the Portuguese colony that published the greatest number of medical journals, with eight. Finally, abroad, four journals were published in Paris, an expression of the cultural links established between the Portuguese intelligentsia and the French capital that from the eighteenth century became the destination of political and intellectual exiles, or simply the place to seek further education and cultural refinement.[32]

To the first category a) (Figure 1) belong the six journals especially focussed on the defence of doctors' professional interests, although other types of medical periodicals also addressed them but not exclusively. With one exception, corporative journals naturally emerged linked to medical professional associations. The Sociedade União Médica (Society Medical Union), founded in Porto, in 1882, and lasting until 1898, the year the Associação dos Médicos Portugueses (Association of Portuguese Physicians) was launched in Lisbon, publishing a bulletin and aiming at representing and defending the profession nationwide, as well as promoting doctors' appearance, standards of living, and social status, especially in the capital.

The very active Associação dos Médicos do Norte de Portugal (Association of Physicians of Northern Portugal), created in Porto, in 1909, after 1911 was renamed Associação Médica Lusitana (Lusitanian Medical Association), also published a bulletin, the latter name showing the aim of representating the profession nationwide and competing with its Lisbon counterpart. The Associação dos Médicos do Centro de Portugal (Association of Physicians of Central Portugal), founded in Coimbra in 1911, tried to launch a national federation of medical associations, which had the agreement of the northern association, but the opposition of Lisbon.

Finally, a private firm with the name União Médica (Medical Union), created in 1911, in Portalegre, southern Portugal, supported the journal with the same name published in the newspaper format. It claimed to defend the interests of provincial doctors whose salaries and working conditions were poor, and who did not feel represented by the former.[33]

Most periodicals in categories b) amounting to five, and c) to 29, have a clear mixed character: not only did they include medical and surgical topics, statistics and medical research, but they also dealt with corporative issues, and focussed on politics, education, medical history, women and child care, eugenics, etc. Especially the independent titles— in the sense they had no formal link to an institution, although their editors and contributors generally held positions in medical schools and hospitals, and were leading members of medical societies and associations—were often closer to a magazine[34] than a journal. This new medium was to emerge in the early twentieth century and 'ushered in the technologizing of information.'[35] Although they varied in format, genres and emphases, when dealing with political, social and corporative issues they used a propagandistic tone, like the MC in Lisbon, and its Porto counterpart, the monthly Medicina Moderna (Modern Medicine, hereafter MM).

Specialized journals in specific medical fields included in d) amounting to 28, and h) amounting to four were normally published by hospitals, and after 1911, also by the faculties of medicine in the three cities, specialized and research institutes, with Lisbon standing out. In the 1880s, specialists became part of the medical academic elite and a recognized social category in Europe,[36] the following pre-conditions being essential to the emergence of specialism: the unification of medicine and surgery, 'a community of scholars built around the research imperative, and institutions organized around a particular notion of administrative rationality.'[37]

In Portugal, the first attempts at specialization also occurred in the 1880s, although were not always successful. For example, the importance that psychiatry and psychiatrists had in those years, and the medicalization of the judicial system characteristic of this period, are evident in generalist journals, published by medical societies and independent bodies such as *MC*, but the specialized journal in the field, the *Revista de Nevrologia e Psichiatria* (*Review of Neurology and Psychiatry*, 1888–1889) was short-lived.[38] Then, the absence of specific courses on neurology and psychiatry in Portuguese medical schools, which prompted psychiatrists to write to *MC* and other periodicals on the need to introduce courses on these disciplines in medical teaching, certainly contributed to making that specialized journal hard to sustain and accounts for its short life. A comparable situation occurred in ophthalmology with two initial attempts at creating a specialized journal, both short-lived (Figure 1). Courses on ophthalmology at the LMSS began only in 1890, delivered by Caetano Gama Pinto (1853–1945), who had been trained and taught in Heidelberg.[39]

Only during the First Republic did specialized periodicals, this time published in the context of faculties of medicine and institutes, succeed, due to their institutional backing within the spirit of the republican reform of higher education promoting scientific research. They testify to the increasing social and political significance of newly established laboratory-based medical disciplines, the generalist medical press and the sessions at medical societies having paved the way for their emergence. Such was the case of bacteriology, tropical medicine, and legal medicine, the respective journals being associated with medical structures established in Lisbon in the early twentieth century, run by doctors trained abroad: the Bacteriological Institute, the School of Tropical Medicine, and the Institute of Legal Medicine. This group comprised also the journals published by the only Portuguese privately funded institute devoted to biomedical research, the Institute Bento da Rocha Cabral established in Lisbon, in 1922,[40] and by the Oncology Institute, in 1923.[41]

Another group of journals is that devoted to statistics (epidemiology, mortality, etc.) included in e), f) and g), amounting respectively to five, nine and 13 journals, which were published by hospitals, city, governmental authorities, and the military, in the three main cities on the mainland and in the colonies. Such periodicals materialized, in Portugal, amidst the growing recognition of statistical thinking as a powerful instrument, throughout the nineteenth century, when statistical patterns came to be seen as explanatory, leading to a new style of reasoning characteristic of modern industrial societies.[42]

As noted before, this was a period that ushered in doctors' commitment to the development of laboratory-based medicine, medical statistics, and biomedical research in Portugal, within a process by which they tried to build up something akin to what Michel Foucault has called 'biopower.' The main aim was the control and management of populations, with emphasis on the protection of life through the regulation of the subject's body, mainly by practices of public health. Groups such as women, children, and individuals considered as a danger to social order could be particularly targeted and the

Portuguese medical press is no exception in this respect.[43] Thus, in the period under consideration, Portuguese doctors were committed not only to the medicalization of the workers, the poor, and the 'feeble minded,' perceived as a threat to social order and public health, but also of women and children, education, culture, and the city.[44] In effect, various leading doctors of this period wrote on these topics, and took part in governmental bodies and committees devoted to education and medical care, as well as in municipalities, notably in Lisbon and Porto.

Periodicals included in k) comprised four journals devoted to the natural sciences in general and biology published in French by scientific societies closely associated with the research school of Athias. Together with his disciples and associates, in addition to establishing in Portugal new biomedical disciplines, notably in the Faculty of Medicine of Lisbon and the Institute Rocha Cabral, they founded learned societies. Such was the case of the Portuguese Society of Natural Sciences and respective journals with the aim of mobilizing scientists and promoting the natural sciences, especially biology and chemistry, with little expression in Portugal outside academia. These disciplines, in addition, constituted the scientific foundations of laboratory-based medicine, and for a long time were locally considered subsidiary to engineering and medicine.

Finally, the categories comprising a small number of journals. Thus, those included in i) published data obtained in commercial laboratories most devoted to clinical tests; in j) to sanitary education such as the bulletin of the Assistência Nacional aos Tuberculosos (National Assistance to Tuberculosis Patients); in l) focussed predominantly on medical history and popularization (also present in the journals included in b) and c) of much wider circulation). The latter certainly contributed to build up a collective memory of medical progress and a Portuguese medical tradition. Homeopathy and similar practices, which were not amenable to the practices and theories of laboratory-based allopathic medicine, had naturally little expression in the medical press as the limited and short-lived number of journals in m) shows. Yearbooks and bibliographic bulletins in n), and directories included in o) provided useful practical information, the latter for both doctors, vets, nurses, and patients; finally, the satirical journals in p) were few and occasional, which does not exclude their interest as expressions through humor of divergent opinions.

Editors, Funding and Readership

The editors of the majority of the medical periodicals were physicians who derived their income from the practice of their profession in medical schools, hospitals, research institutes, private clinical practice and laboratories, and the same applies to the redactors. Both contributed articles not only to the periodical to which they were formally linked, by focussing on medical and surgical topics, but also by writing in a journalistic and propagandistic style on politics, education, culture and society[45] in medical periodicals of a more overtly mixed character (types b) and c)), and in the general press.[46] Most doctors were part of networks, which naturally differ from the networks of journalists or women authors as addressed in the literature on periodical studies,[47] who made a living out of writing, be it novels, serials and/or articles for the periodical press. Despite the rivalries opposing Lisbon, Coimbra and Porto and respective institutions, networks had a national character by linking doctors operating in the three cities, and an international dimension through contacts they had abroad. From the perspective of the medical press alone, in addition to the networks composed of editors, printers, authors, illustrators and photographers, still to be unraveled, the Portuguese Association of the Medical Press (PAMP) and the International Association of the Medical Press (IAMP) were themselves national and international networks of medical periodicals, editors and authors.

Little is known about the number of copies each journal printed, their distribution and how they were funded as well as their price and number of subscribers; so far only the price of the Portuguese journals represented in the IAMP is known: between the affordable sums of 2,000 and 3,000 *reis* (10 to 20 French francs) for the annual subscription.[48]

Medical journals associated with teaching or research institutions were funded by their budgets, and normally exchanged periodicals with other institutions, both in Portugal and abroad, which explains why some Portuguese periodicals were written in French to facilitate a two-way circulation. Journals published by professional associations and learned societies were naturally paid by membership fees and advertisements on medical drugs and instruments. Journals like the *Boletim da Associação dos Medicos Portuguezes* (Bulletin of the Association of Portuguese Physicians), however, also included advertisements on automobiles, clothing, and other items thought of as especially suited for doctors that were also a sign of their growing status in the main cities.

Although one does not know for sure the reasons that may account for the public and doctors subscribing to these journals, in the case of the latter it is plausible to think of various explanations: from a wish to update their knowledge to a commitment to social and political causes, or simply more prosaic motives. Volumes of a medical journal, especially among those included in b) and c) could be a sign of distinction to be displayed on the shelves of the living room in a doctor's home, or in the office, or even in the waiting room at the private practice, where the bourgeois patient could read them. As Dillane showed in the case of George Eliot's decision to publish her historical novel *Romola* in serial form in *Cornhill Magazine*, in 1862, the 'attention to the affective constitutes attention to genre, network, audience, and the politics of aesthetics'[49] and also applies to articles in medical journals included in the above categories. A certain voyeurism and mixed emotions between curiosity and repulsion caused by descriptions or images of certain medical conditions, together with serialized reports on crimes and their medical interpretation, resorted to affect, often bordering on the chap-book, were bound to catch the attention of patients, doctors, their wives, families and circles of friends, adding to the number of readers.

Overall, the Portuguese medical press in this period has naturally to be assessed bearing in mind the country's demography, the number of doctors and the high rates of illiteracy. The population on mainland Portugal grew from c.3,5000,000 people in 1870, to c.5,500,000 in 1910. The rate of illiteracy was c.80% between 1878 and 1900, decreasing to c.70–65% between 1911 and 1930;[50] as to the number of doctors nationwide little is known, seemingly 2,000 in the 1880s,[51] but they increased with time, especially during and after the First Republic.

In this context, the character of the Portuguese publishing apparatus necessarily entailed a certain degree of fictionalization of audiences, a kind of Lippmann's 'phantom public,'[52] and an immense faith in the transformative capacity of the press, propaganda and education. The gap between intended and actual audiences[53] is even more striking as outside the urban bourgeoisie the population was obviously held to oral communication rather than written, the main spaces of sociability being taverns and the religious services of the Roman Catholic Church, the latter representing a power that the medical press was fully committed to counteract.

It is thus unlikely that Portuguese medical journals of this period were profitable commercial ventures or expected to be profitable in a strict sense, but only a systematic survey on the inclusion of advertisements, publication costs, and subscriptions would allow for more definitive claims. It seems that their publication, however, was rather a matter of legitimating the medical profession, creating a socio-cultural elite, propagating a faith in medicine, science and the republic, and educating the nation's spirit in order to sustain the regime and achieve progress. Doctors' motives corroborate Judt's view that 'men are motivated by what they think and believe and not just by objective and measurable interest (…). But interest, belief and emotion are not inherently incompatible sources of human behaviour.'[54]

The Weekly A Medicina Contemporânea

The first issue of *MC* was published in 1883. Primarily addressed to doctors, but readable by anybody with a modicum of instruction and knowledge of general culture, this 'newspaper,' as it was then called, was meant to: 'report on the recent scientific advancements made abroad; emphasise studies carried out in Portugal; advocate all useful reforms regarding medicine and its practice,' and lead doctors, as citizens, to react against the 'numbness of their fellow citizens.'[55]

The Founders

A group of physicians all teaching at the LMSS, and leading members of the nationwide influential Lisbon Society of Medical Sciences (Sociedade das Ciências Medicas, hereafter LSMS) founded *MC*. They were Manuel Bento de Sousa (1835–1899), José Tomás de Sousa Martins (1843–1897), and Miguel Bombarda (1851–1910), accompanied by a group of distinguished colleagues who often contributed articles, the redactors.

MC's first director was Bombarda, a former graduate from the LMSS, and since 1880 professor of physiology and histology. A cultured man aware of the main medical issues and debates taking place in Europe and the USA, he was an evolutionist, monist, materialist,[56] and anticlerical, especially anti-Jesuit like most republicans. An advocate of the organic basis of mental illness, he specialized in psychiatry. A Freemason inclined to utopian socialism, he became Member of Parliament in 1908, and in 1909 part of a revolutionary committee aimed at overthrowing the monarchy. Although he had never practised laboratory research, Bombarda became fully committed to preaching laboratory-based medicine, campaigning for the construction of important medical and laboratory facilities in Lisbon, and supporting younger doctors who had trained abroad following their return to Portugal.

He introduced radical changes in the organization of medical services, teaching and research in the LMSS and the psychiatric hospital (Hospital de Rilhafoles) that was later named after him.[57] As its director, from 1892 he implemented a complete reorganization based on the division of patients according to sex and their distribution according to categories.[58] Caring for mental patients became in this way 'technologized:' they were kept clean and properly fed, and an administrative system was established in the hospital according to which records and clinical notes had to be kept so patients could be monitored on a regular basis and conclusions derived regarding symptoms, and the approaches and methods used in treating them.[59] Bombarda abolished repressive practices within the hospital and replaced them with medical and occupational therapies; he also advocated the inclusion of the inimputability of mental patients in the legislation. Bombarda lectured doctors and medical students on psychiatry on Sundays, paving the way for the creation of the respective chair in 1911, at the FML.

Bombarda was an advocate of preventive eugenics, notably by controlling marriage and reproduction, and claimed the need to legislate on this matter, but as he put it, only after the Portuguese had been persuaded of this necessity by propaganda.[60] He coordinated the scientific committee advising the team of architects behind the construction of the new impressive building of the LMSS inaugurated in 1906, and the organization of the 15th Meeting of the International Medical Congress and of the IAMP held in Lisbon on the occasion.

On 3 October 1910, the very eve of the monarchy being overthrown, a former mental patient assassinated Bombarda. Not even his dead body escaped from scientific scrutiny, as detailed and realistic reports of the surgery and autopsy performed on him were published in MC.[61] Such an energetic man was, according to the autopsy, destined to die sooner rather than later not by God's will, or at the hands of a lunatic, but from the failure of vital organs. They were too damaged to allow recovery from the surgery carried out to extract the bullets shortly after the shooting.

Martins, another founder of MC, had graduated in medicine from the LMSS in 1868, where he came to teach pathology, semiology, and the history of medicine. A renowned local expert on tuberculosis, which then reached almost epidemic proportions in Lisbon,[62] he became honorary doctor of the Royal Household and the Government, and was admired for caring for impoverished patients for free. Martins is associated with the conversion of Serra da Estrela, the Portuguese highest mountain, into the 'magic mountain' where patients would seek a cure. Suffering himself from tuberculosis and a heart condition, both causing him great pain, he took his own life by resorting to a morphine injection. Like Charles Richet and Arthur Conan Doyle who entertained a correspondence on psychic phenomena, Martins was a spiritualist.[63] Following his death, spiritualists and common people 'canonized' him; his statue, inaugurated in 1907 in front of the new buildings of the LMSS, was turned ironically into a shrine where, to this day, people pray and give thanks for his alleged miraculous cures.

Finally, Sousa, the elder of MC's founding trio, was professor of surgery and anatomy at the LMSS.[64] He became known for his investigations on the gustatory function of the Wrisberg nerve in 1870, and as the organizer of the 1st National Congress of Medicine in 1898, the main themes of the meeting being tuberculosis, and maternal and child health, as in both cases mortality was unacceptably high in Portugal.[65] As MC's literary editor and writer, Sousa adopted the pen-name Marcos Pinto. He turned to full-time journalism in later life, as he had always preferred writing to clinical practice.

Sousa, Bombarda and Martins were at the origin of two medical-journalistic tra-ditions, according to Mira, a distinguished researcher and doctor-journalist of the 'Gener-ation of 1911.' In his view, Bombarda epitomized the pamphleteer brand who thrilled his audiences and mobilized them; Martins, in turn, with the gift of gab and being 'naturally eloquent,' like Bombarda played with emotion, his style being most successful among medical students, colleagues and lay audiences. In contrast, Sousa partook of a sober style, ascribed to his personality and upbringing as an adopted child of a noble family.[66] He was said to combine aristocratic manners with a satirical and controversialist vein expressed in articles and books such as *Doutor Minerva* (*Doctor Minerva*), a satire on the teaching methods in Portuguese schools, and *A Parvónia* (*Silly Land*), a caricature of Lisbon mores and parochialism, in which he also satirized the press.[67] Sousa's colleagues revered him, but with a pinch of criticism. Bombarda commented on his alleged pessimism and inertia as the result of the 'powerful influence of a hypochondriac nature, an evident fault in his portentous mental machinery.'[68] But to the well-travelled 'Generation of 1911,' Sousa incarnated in his 'aristocratic reserve' their most cherished virtues—depth, sobriety, wit, elegant writing, and a kind of prudent distance regarding the latest novelty, usually uncritically and hastily embraced by his peers.[69]

MC's Format, Layout, Structure and Contents

The weekly *MC* mixed the characteristics of a medical journal and a newspaper, these features converging to make it something close to a magazine.[70] Each issue was published in the format 22×31cm, usually comprised of around eight pages numbered consecutively from one issue to the next, as they were supposed to be bound annually in a single volume. The annual volume had a front page (Figure 2) followed by a table of contents for the whole year, organized into sections. Articles were printed in two columns; the font size was around eight or smaller, when presenting statistics and legislation. The quality of the paper and ink was variable.

Issues had no cover until 1888; from then onwards the cover was used to print adver-tisements.[71] Prior to these, in 1886 *MC* published an early form of advertisement, the 'Ates-tados Médicos' (literally medical statements), placed at the end of an issue. They were written by Spanish doctors on behalf of the firm Scott & Brown, New York, which sold pala-table codfish oil, certainly seeking to expand its business to the whole Iberian Peninsula. These statements were a source of income to the journal, not to mention to the physicians who wrote them, but for unknown reasons in subsequent years they vanished for good. In the 1920s, advertisements appeared inside the journal. From mineral water, toothpaste, and milk powder, to a variety of drugs, these items had the implicit approval of the most distinguished doctors in the capital.

MC was funded by subscriptions and advertisements, but at least initially presumably by contributions from those involved in its publication, who were motivated by a commit-ment to professional, social and political causes. *MC*'s annual subscription amounted to 3,000 *reis* (20 French francs) and abroad 4,000 *reis*.

The use of images was generally scarce, likely to reduce costs. Initially, engravings were printed, usually representing the anatomy of a body part; buildings and plans of buildings; or a portrait of a recently deceased doctor in the respective obituary. The

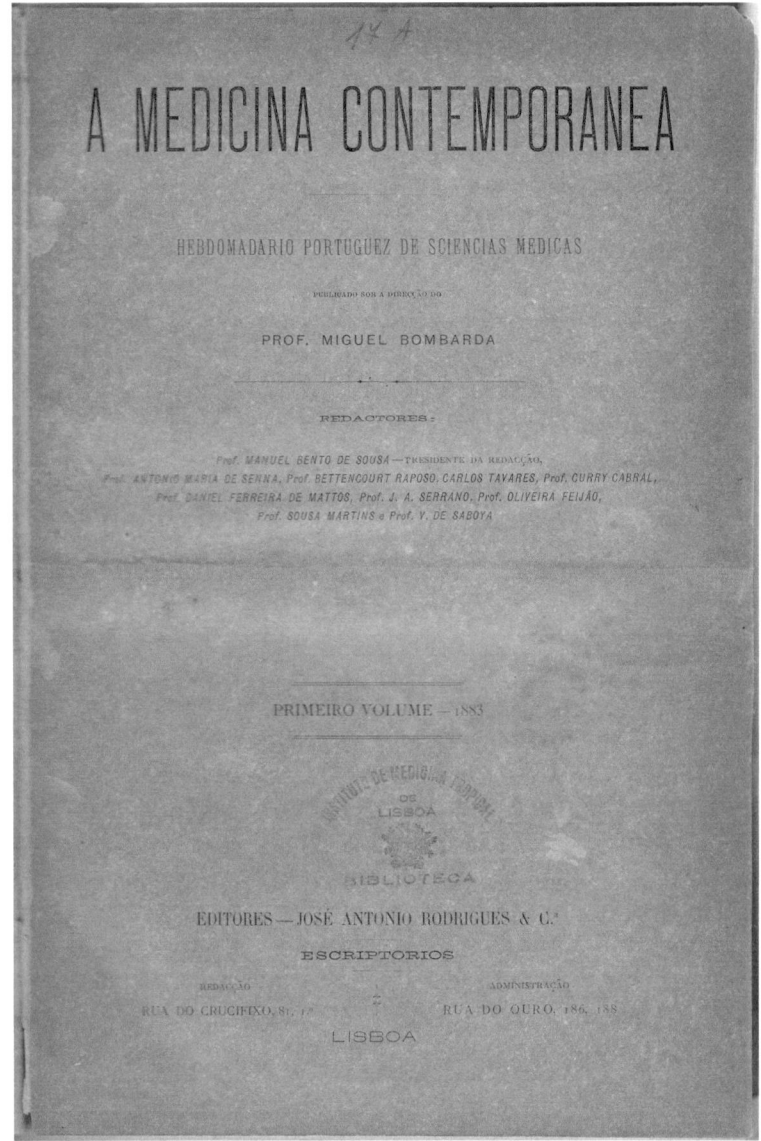

FIGURE 2
Front page of the 1st annual volume of the journal A Medicina Contemporânea 1 (1883)

drawings, which accompanied the series of articles on mental illness published by António Senna (1845–1890)—a renowned psychiatrist, who had attended Charcot's and Brown-Séquard's courses in Paris, member of the committee that assisted Bombarda in reorganizing the Rilhafoles Hospital, and of *MC*'s redaction[72] —are particularly striking in number and kind. They displayed what was usually kept out of sight in hospital and prison dungeons, or shamefully hidden in a bourgeois residence: the mental patient, the inadequate spaces of a psychiatric hospital, straitjackets, and other paraphernalia (Figure 3)—resorting

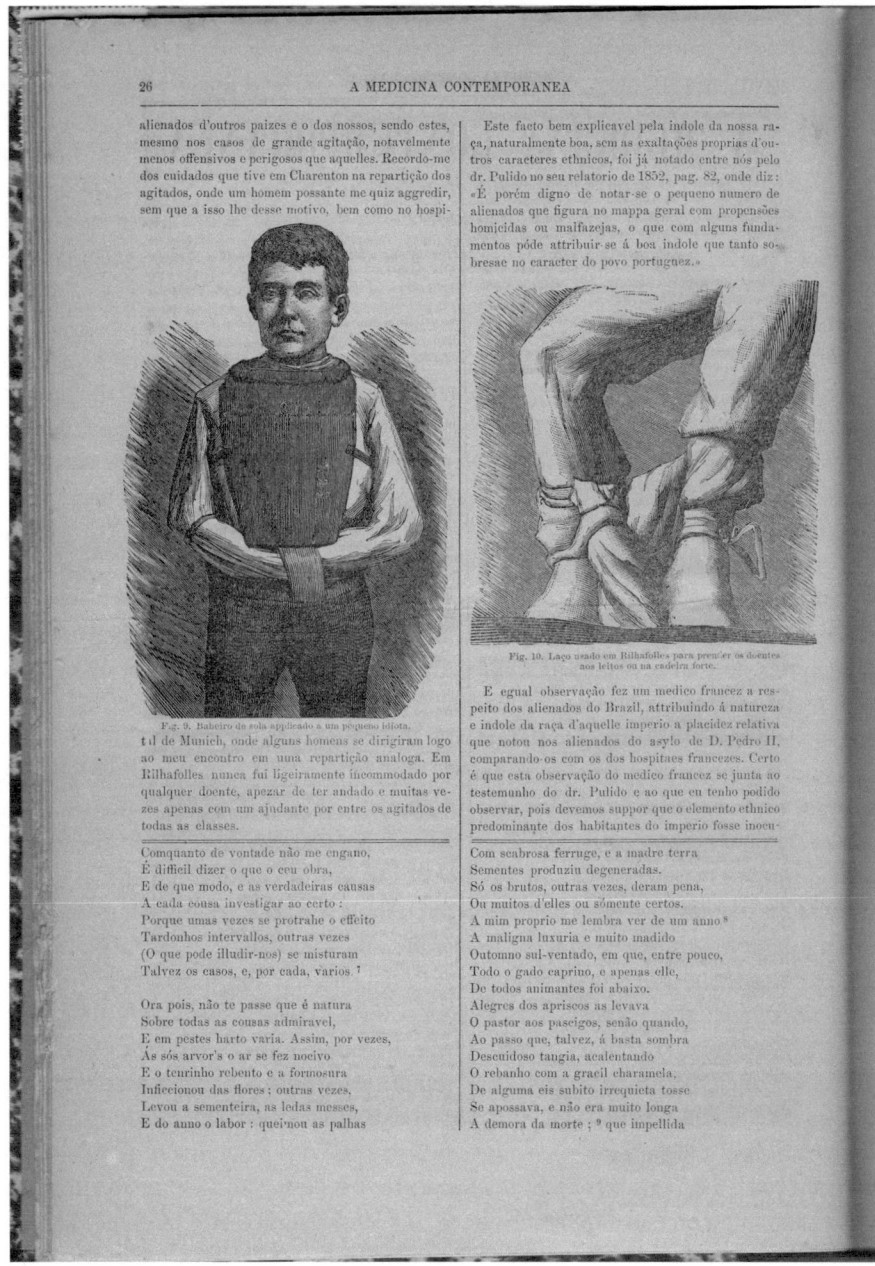

FIGURE 3
Straitjacket applied to a young idiot; Loop used at Rilhafoles Hospital to tie patients to beds and special chairs. António Maria de Senna, "Os Alienados em Portugal." Medicina Contemporânea 2 (1884): 26

to affect, but within limits that photography would erase for the sake of 'realism' and 'objectivity.'[73] Photography made its first appearance in *MC* in the image of a microscopic preparation in 1899, and a picture of a (crane-encephalic) X-ray was first printed in 1900.[74]

Although many issues began with a signed serialized piece of original research, often an untitled and unsigned editorial note replaced it. Normally, editorials had marked ideological and political content such as this published in 1884: 'It is huge the influence doctors have on populations, especially in small localities, but opposite influences and political dependence are equally huge, which force doctors to intervene in electoral fights and have an active role in attaining objectives immediately beneficial.'[75] Similarly, in the politically eventful year of 1910, one reads an account of the recent elections in Lisbon: 'Civic education in Lisbon was achieved by the propaganda voiced by the freedom coryphaeus, first of all the republican party ... people have realized that under the present rule [the monarchy] all guaranties of freedom and morality have failed.'[76]

Articles devoted to original research were occasionally a serialized critical compilation of articles published in foreign journals. Serials had become fashionable in Portuguese literary circles in the 1860s,[77] and *MC*'s redactors likewise adopted this form consistently, with a similar purpose: to establish a contract with readers, by anticipating what they wanted,[78] or what they were led to want. The poetic form was also used, an example being a translation of Girolamo Frascatoro's Latin poem entitled 'Syphilis,' also serialized, this infection being naturally a recurrent theme.[79]

Digests of international medical literature on particular drugs, or news on medical meetings were also serialized. *MC* also informed doctors of positions available nationwide and reported on Parliamentary discussions on hygienic problems, especially affecting Lisbon. Short news of a lighter nature but with the greatest effect in showing that medicine was definitely being 'aristocratized' were also included: 'A Medical Prince.—The German press reports that Ludwig Ferdinand von Bayern, of the House of Wittelsbach, has just graduated from the Faculty of Medicine, in Munich. He is the second who has studied medicine.'[80] Finally, every issue usually ended with a weekly statistical bulletin, containing a table with the sanitary statistics of the main European cities, including Lisbon.

All sorts of questions were addressed through the pages of *MC*, usually from a Lisbon perspective: medical teaching and education, the situation of general and psychiatric hospitals;[81] the rejection of nuns in hospital nursing, eugenics, and tuberculosis—the main reason underlying the spread of this illness being 'the moral degeneration of the people.'[82] In addition, Lisbon's hygiene, tropical medicine, the First World War and the organization of medical services in various countries were also object of special attention. *MC*'s counterpart in Porto, however, the monthly *MM*, despite its director's ideological affinities with his *MC* colleagues—when he claimed that 'science is the true Messiah, the single redemptor of Man on this planet,' in the utopia for the 20th century that he published in 1924[83]—imprinted on *MM* a different stance. The journal aimed at representing northern Portugal, with its small towns, remote villages, and deprived places, rather than simply Porto, then a burgeoning city undergoing demographic, urban, economic and cultural expansion.[84]

Since the inaugural editorial note published in January 1883, medical education and training became a recurring and major theme in *MC*, as well as in the comparisons of Portugal with other European countries, Germany becoming a role model in this respect. However, the insistence on the reform of medical teaching had an implicit purpose: controlling the access to the profession, with the physicians teaching in the capital setting the norm. Skirmishes opposing Lisbon- and Porto- to Coimbra-based professors of medicine were recurrent in *MC* until 1911, with the former claiming for the extinction of the FMUC in 1885,[85] accused of poor standards that allegedly had caused a drastic decrease in the number of students.[86]

Primary and secondary education was equally the object of much criticism, from schools' cobwebbed buildings to the kind of gymnastics practiced by pupils.[87] Almost a disease, education in Portugal would be only curable by using a single prescription: a 'rigorous and positive scientific education,' which 'from the cradle must be relentless and regularly delivered every day,' as it was 'the single origin of progress and social enhancement.' [88]

Corporative issues were naturally a permanent concern in *MC*: doctors' demarcation from charlatans, wages, social status, and prerogatives. Since the 1880s, doctors' municipal- or government-derived income had been very modest, especially in the provinces, and the health systems of professional mutual associations paid them low and variable wages. This situation explains why, as early as 1884, an *MC* editorial note discussed the need for reform of the Portuguese electoral system so as to include representatives of the medical profession.[89] Despite the presence of a number of physicians in the bicameral political system, the question of having a physician elected in Parliament as a representative of the profession was raised.[90] In effect, in the National Constituent Assembly of 1911, devoted to the task of writing the constitution for the First Republic, which chose for its official motto 'Health and Fraternity,' [91] physicians reached the summit and had the largest number of seats (22.7%) among the nation's representatives.[92]

Concluding Remarks

Between the 1880s and 1926, in Europe and Portugal, the social and political ascendance of medical doctors coincided with the development of laboratory-based medicine and research, the emergence of a mass press, and consequently the medical press coming to be perceived as a powerful instrument of professional, social, cultural, and political change. Locally, this process also coincided with the republican movements in which a number of doctors took part, and the growing importance of Lisbon as the nation's scientific, medical and cultural capital, then seeking to attain the standards of a European metropolis.

By approaching the massive Portuguese publishing apparatus as it pertains to the medical press—with regard to the size of the medical community, the country's population, and the high rate of illiteracy—Portuguese physicians emerge as the untiring organizers of the profession and, through propaganda, also of 'public opinion,' as the analysis of the journal *Medicina Contemporânea* has shown. In this way, the publishing apparatus was bound to generate what Lippmann, in his reflections on the democratic system, called a 'phantom public.' The disproportion between agents (the physicians) and bystanders (the potential readers) was huge, particularly outside the main cities. Especially in Porto and Lisbon, however, many of these journals created the possibility of a dialogue among doctors and between them, their inhabitants and political decision-makers, which materialized in the construction and/or reorganization of medical and research structures.

Portuguese doctors of this period can thus be described by what Gramsci—who like Lippmann lived precisely in this period—called 'organic intellectuals' in his reflections on the importance of ideology and conceptualization of the role of intellectuals. Until the end of the First Republic in 1926, especially in Lisbon, physicians, the republic, and the city all converged and reinforced each other in creating 'hegemony' by constituting what Gramsci called a 'historic bloc.'[93] In Porto, a similar process occurred, but with the intention of the city becoming representative of northern Portugal, a notion that often included central Portugal, as the University of Coimbra was allegedly losing its traditional political influence in the formation of the Portuguese intelligentsia.

But when reflecting on the role of propaganda and the medicalization of various areas of individual and social life, as well as the concomitant creation or reorganization of institutions such as hospitals, laboratories and schools, Ellul's concept of propaganda as a sociological phenomenon entwined in a society increasingly dominated by 'technique' comes to mind.[94] The interest of Portuguese doctors in education, in addition, as if it were a question of public health was motivated by their intent of molding people's minds, a prerequisite of propaganda. The Portuguese medical press as a propaganda apparatus was thus supposed not only to propagate medical knowledge and techniques in the medical community, but also to generate a public sphere, in which topics could be debated within a shared ideological framework, in order to 'manufacture consent'[95] and in this way ensure the sustainability of the republic.

It is unlikely that the main aim of the Portuguese medical publishing apparatus was profit, which does not exclude the possibility of a small number of medical journals paid by membership subscriptions and advertising being profitable, at least for a while, but further research is required to substantiate more definitive claims. If the medical publishing apparatus were overall a lucrative enterprise, it could be amenable to Herman's and Chomsky's 'propaganda model,' but naturally, there are fundamental differences given the distinct contexts.[96] The Portuguese medical press was not concentrated in the hands of a media corporation or a conglomerate like in the 'propaganda model,' but of an increasingly powerful professional group. Its chief aim was the propagation of an ideology believed to be capable of generating a new reality: creating a market for a new breed of technically competent and highly cultured physicians and surgeons, who were the elite of the republic; promoting a healthy, educated and prosperous republican society, sharing in the scientifically based culture propagated by the medical profession.

Acknowledgements

This research was carried out in the context of CIUHCT (Interuniversity Centre for the History of Science and Technology), which is funded by Fundação para a Ciência e a Tecnologia (UID/HIS/00286/2013). The authors wish thank the anonymous referees for their comments and criticism, and to Jennifer Wallis and Sally Frampton for their always kind assistance and linguistic suggestions. A word of gratitude also goes to André Pereira for his technical assistance.

Disclosure statement

No potential conflict of interest was reported by the authors.

Funding

This research was carried out in the context of CIUHCT (Interuniversity Centre for the History of Science and Technology), which is funded by Fundação para a Ciência e a Tecnologia (UID/HIS/00286/2013).

Notes

1. Paulo, *Periódicos* and Athias, *Catálogo*.
2. Van Remoortel et al. "Joining Forces," 1–3.
3. The digital form poses problems to the field of periodical studies and history, which has been amply discussed in the literature. van Remoortel et al. "Joinig Forces," 1–3; Lathan and Sholes, "The Rise," 517–31; Ardis, "Towards a Theory;" Brake, "On Print Culture," 125–36; Allen, "Lost and Now Found;" Fyfe, "An Archaeology," 564–77.
4. Latham and Sholes "The Rise," 517.
5. Steel and Broersma, "Redefining," 235–7.
6. Tengarrinha, *História*, 191–201 and Sousa et al. eds. *Pensamento*, 16–51
7. Regarding science and medicine in newspapers see Simões, Carneiro, Diogo, "Riding the Wave" and Almeida, *Saúde*.
8. The Portuguese obviously do not constitute a race, but this was the term then used.
9. Together with *Jornal da Sociedade de Ciências Médicas, Bulletin da Associação dos Médicos Portugueses, Archivos d'Hygiene e Patología Exoticas,* and *Polytechnia,* all published in Lisbon; *Movimento Medico,* published in Coimbra, and *Porto Medico,* in Porto. N. A. *Association Internationale.*
10. Amaral, "A Geração de 1911."
11. Mergoupi-Savaidou, Papanelopoulo, Carneiro, "Popularization," 966–77; Papanelopoulo, Nieto-Galan and Perdiguero, eds., *Popularizing.*
12. Topham, "Historicizing," 310–8; Hilgartner, "The Dominant View," 519–39; Porter, *Popularization*; Michaels, "Medical Propaganda," 159–78.
13. Occasionally the term 'vulgarização' (vulgarisation) appears as an equivalent.
14. Lippmann's expression in Public Opinion.
15. Carneiro and Amaral, "Propaganda," 138–66.
16. Ramos, "A Formação," 483–528; Fernandes, "Aspectos," 335–40.
17. Amaral, "The Emergence."
18. Quental, *Causas.*
19. Cunningham and Williams, eds., *Laboratory.*
20. Luz, "A Propagação," 239–432; Carneiro et al."Geology," 331–54.
21. Abbott, *System of Professions.*
22. Ramos, "A Formação," 499.
23. Amaral, "The Emergence."
24. *Paul, Sorcerer's.*
25. Amaral, "The Emergence," and Carneiro and Amaral, "Propaganda."
26. Nieto-Galan, "Antonio Gramsci," 453–78; Sassoon, "The People," 137–68; Lears, "The Concept," 567–9.
27. A feature of propaganda according to Ellul. Ellul, *Propaganda,* 70 and 214.

28. On the complexities of defining periodicals, see Philpotts, "Defining."
29. The FMUC was the only to give the title of doctor; graduates from the LMSS and PMSS were called Mr., but they could be appointed for medical positions on par with Coimbra graduates.
30. Carneiro and Amaral, "Propaganda," 140.
31. Doctors trained in India were not allowed to practice medicine on mainland Portugal.
32. Carneiro, Simões, Diogo, "Enlightenment Science," 591–619; Reis, "Scientific Dissemination," 83–118.
33. Only in 1933, during Salazar dictatorship, was a single medical professional association created, operating nationwide to this day, the Ordem dos Médicos. Reis, *História da Ordem*, 19–50–118.
34. On magazines, see Latham, "The Mess."
35. Lathan, "Affordance."
36. Weisz, "The Emergence," 536–75.
37. Ibid.
38. Pereira, "A Evolução," 365–68. The director was António Bettencoturt Rodrigues (1854–1933) who had graduated in medicine in Paris and worked with Jean-Martin Charcot.
39. Ibid.
40. Carneiro & Amaral, "Propaganda".
41. Both published by the Institute Rocha Cabral the *Travaux de Laboratoire* aimed at the international scientific community and *Actualidades Biológicas* for a national educated but not specialized readership. The *Arquivo de Patologia* was associated with cancer research.
42. Hacking, *Taming*.
43. Foucault, *Naissance de la Biopolitique* and Gougelet, "The World," 43–66.
44. Conrad, "Medicalization;" Crawford, "Healthism."
45. It is worth mentioning that doctors, especially belonging to the Generation of 1911, appropriated these themes and wrote on them in the general press, in addition to the medical periodicals.
46. Bearing in mind that most periodicals are heterogeneous, as Latham and Sholes, and Green have emphasised. Latham and Sholes, "The Rise," Green, "Around 1910."
47. Brake, "Time's Turbulence," 115–27; Easley, "Victorian Networks," 111–4; Fagg, Pethers, Vandome. "Networks," 93–104; Murphy, "Visualizing Networks," iii–xv.
48. *Reis*, then Portuguese currency. *Association Internationale*, 65–8.
49. Dilanne, "Forms of Affect," 11.
50. Marques, *História*, vol.2, 31 and 185–6.
51. According to the editorial note *MC* 2 (1884): 121.
52. Lippmann, *Phantom Public* and *Public Opinion*.
53. Mergoupi-Savaidou, Papanelopoulou, & Carneiro, "Popularization."
54. Judt, *When the Facts*, 78–9.
55. [Untitled and unsigned editorial note], MC 1 (1883), 2.
56. Bombarda's brands of monism and materialism are analysed in Barata-Moura "Miguel Bombarda," 61.
57. The psychiatric Hospital Miguel Bombarda was equipped with a panopticum in 1896, and its architecture has features, which became common only in the 1920s and 30s.
58. Cintra, ed., *Miguel*, 42–43.

59. Cintra, ed., Miguel; Fernandes, *A Psiquiatria*, and Madureira, "A Estatística," 283–303.
60. Bombarda, "Degenerescência," 217–8; Pereira, *Darwin*, 550–2.
61. Amado et al. "Miguel," 321–30.
62. Vieira, *Conhecer*.
63. Pais, *Sousa Martins*.
64. Cabral, *Elogio*.
65. In 1900, in Portugal one in five children would die in infancy, and one pregnant woman in 100 would die in childbirth. Regarding tuberculososis, the rate in 1898 was 297–396 TB patients in 100,000 inhabitants. Alves, *A Faculdade*, 67–69
66. Sousa was a baby orphan when the Count of Murça adopted him.
67. Sousa, *A Parvónia*.
68. Bombarda, quoted in Mira, *Manuel*, 183.
69. Mira, *Manuel*, 181–182.
70. Mussell, "The Matter"
71. Monteiro argued that advertisements in *MC* appeared in the first decade of the 20th century, which is not exact. Monteiro *A Medicina*, 25–29.
72. This series was later published in book form, in 1885. Sena, *Os Alienados*.
73. Daston & Galison, "Image."
74. Bombarda, "Epilepsia," 187. Image very blurred.
75. [Untitled and unsigned editorial note] *MC* 2 (1884): 121.
76. [Presumably Bombarda] "Eleições," 281.
77. Ramos, "A formação da *intelligentsia*," 490.
78. Mussell, "The Matter" and Miller, "Genre," 151–67.
79. N.A. "Folhetim: A Syphilis," 1.
80. N.A. "Um Principe," 31.
81. Raposo, "Hospitaes," 40–42.
82. 'A degenerescência moral do povo português como factor de expansão da tuberculose,' name of a session of the meeting 3° Congresso da Liga Nacional contra a Tuberculose, Coimbra, 21–24 April, 1904, the chairman being Bombarda.
83. Castro, *A Felicidade*, 60.
84. Cardoso, "Sociedade," 123–152.
85. "Conselho Superior d'Instrução Pública. Relatorios dos Delegados das Escolas Médicas de Lisboa e Porto,"*MC* 5 (1885), 317–8; 325–8; 333–40; 342–4; 344–7.
86. It is hard to tell whether this claim is sound. Although the number of students that graduated per year from the LMSS is known, similar information for Coimbra and Porto requires further investigation.
87. [Untitled and unsigned editorial notes] *MC* 1 (1883): 147–50; *MC* 2 (1884): 73–4.
88. [Untitled and unsigned editorial notes] *MC* 2 (1884): 49–50.
89. [Untitled and unsigned editorial notes] *MC* 2 (1884): 121.
90. Jorge, [Printed letter addressed to the journal], 129.
91. This motto was used in official documents and correspondence. Alves, "Saúde," 111 and Garnel "Médicos," 230.
92. This was the largest professional category, more than army and navy officers (19.7%) and lawyers and magistrates (17.9%). Graça, "Diferenciação," and Garnel, "Médicos," 230–57.
93. Sassoon, "The People," 154.

94. Ellul's technique is more than machine technology and refers to any complex of standardized means for attaining a pre-defined goal achieved through deliberate and rationalized behavior. Merton, Robert K. "Foreword." In Ellul, *Technological Society*, VI.
95. Lippman, *Public Opinion*, 248.
96. Herman and Chomsky, "Manufacturing."

Bibliography

Abbott, Andrew. *The System of Professions. An Essay on the Division of Expert Labor*. Chicago: University of Chicago Press, 1988.

Allen, Rob. "Lost and Now Found: The Search for the Hidden and Forgotten." *M/C–A Journal of Media and Culture* 20, no. 5 (2017). Accessed 2 November, 2017. http://journal.media-culture.org.au/index.php/mcjournal/article/view/1290.

Almeida, Maria Antónia. *Saúde Pública e Higiene na Imprensa Diária em Anos de Epidemias, 1854–1918*. Lisbon: Edições Colibri, 2013.

Alves, Augusto Lobo. "Congresso dos Médicos Mutualistas. Relatórios." *MC* 13 (1910): 97–100.

Alves, Jorge. "Saúde e Fraternidade. A Saúde Pública na I República." *Corpo. Estado, Medicina e Sociedade no tempo da I República* Lisboa, CNCCR/INCM (2010): 111–129.

Alves, Manuel V. *A Faculdade de Medicina da Universidade de Lisboa. Um Olhar sobre a sua História*. Lisbon: Gradiva, 2011, 67–69.

Amaral, Isabel. "The emergence of new scientific disciplines in Portuguese medicine: Marck Athias's histophysiology research school, Lisbon (1897–1946)." *Annals of Science* 63 (2006): 85–110.

Amaral, Isabel. "A Geração de 1911." In *Médicos e Sociedade – para uma História da Medicina em Portugal no século XX*, edited by António Barros Veloso, Luiz Damas Mora, and Henrique Leitão, 157–172. Lisbon: By the Book, 2017.

Ardis, Ann. "Towards a Theory of Periodical Studies." Accessed 8 November, 2015. https://magmods.wordpress.com/2012/12/28/mla-roundtable-paper-2-defining-the-thick-journal-periodical-codes-and-common-habitus/.

Athias, Marck. *Catálogo das Obras da Colecção Portuguesa de 1825 a 1910*. Lisboa: Faculdade de Medicina (Biblioteca), 1952.

Barata-Moura, José. "Miguel Bombarda e o Materialismo." In *Pensar a Cultura Portuguesa — Homenagem ao Prof. Doutor Francisco José da Gama Caeiro*, edited by Joaquim C. Gonçalves, 167–206. Lisboa: Edições Colibri, 1993.

Bombarda, Miguel. "Degenerescência da Raça." *MC* 3, no. 2 (1900): 217–218.

Bombarda, Miguel. "Epilepsia Traumatica." *MC* 3, no. 2 (1900): 186–187.

Brake, Laurel. "On Print Culture: The State We're In." *Journal of Victorian Culture* 6 (2001): 125–136.

Brake, Laurel. "Time's Turbulence: Mapping Journalism Networks." *Victorian Periodicals Review* 44, no. 2 (2011): 115–127.

Cabral, José Curry. *Elogio Histórico do Professor Manoel Bento de Souza*. Lisboa: Typographia do Dia, 1899.

Cardoso, Duarte. "Sociedade de Instrução do Porto." *Douro* 16 (2003): 123–152.

Carneiro, Ana, et al. "Geology and Religion in Portugal." *Notes & Records of the Royal Society* 67 (2013): 331–354.

Carneiro, Ana, and Isabel Amaral. "Propaganda and Philanthropy: The Institute Bento da Rocha Cabral, the Lisbon Site of Biochemistry (1925–1953)." *Ambix* 62, no. special issue (2015): 138–166.

Carneiro, Ana, Ana Simões, and Maria Paula Diogo. "Enlightenment Science in Portugal: the Estrangeirados and their Communication Networks." *Social Studies of Science* 30 (2000): 591–619.

Castro, António. *A Felicidade no Século XX*. Porto: A. J. O. Castro, 1924.

Cintra, Pedrop, ed. *Miguel Bombarda, Preservar a Memória*. Lisbon: Casa das Letras, 2013.

Conrad, P. "Medicalization and Social Control." *Annual Review of Sociology* 18 (1992): 209–232.

Crawford, R. "Healthism and the Medicalization of Everyday Life." *Health* 10 (1980): 401–420.

Cunningham, Andrew, and Perry Williams, eds. In *The Laboratory Revolution in Medicine*. Cambridge: Cambridge University Press, 1992.

Daston, Lorraine, and Peter Galison. "The Image of Objectivity." *Representations* 40 (1992): 81–128.

Dillane, Fionnuala. "Forms of Afftect, Relationality and Periodical Encounters or 'Pine-Apple for the Million.'." *Journal of European Periodical Studies* 1, no. 1 (Summer 2016): 5–24.

Easley, Alexis. "Victorian Networks and the Periodical Press." *Victorian Periodicals Review* 44, no. 2 (2011): 111–114.

Easley, Alexis, Andrew King, and John Morton, eds. *Researching the Nineteenth-Century Periodical Press: Case Studies*. London: Routledge, 2017.

Ellul, Jacques. *The Technological Society (English translation by John Wilkinson)*. New York: Vintage Books, 1964.

Ellul, Jacques. *Propaganda. The Formation of Men's Attitudes (English translation by Konrad Kellen and Jean Lerner)*. New York: Vintage Books, 1973.

Fagg, John, Matthew Pethers, and Robin Vandome. "Networks and the Nineteenth-Century Periodical." *American Periodicals* 23, no. 2 (2013): 93–104.

Fernandes, H. Barahona. *A Psiquiatria em Portugal*. Lisbon: Roche, 1984.

Fernandes, Ângela. "Aspectos da Retórica de Decadência no Portugal Contemporâneo de Oliveira Martins." *Revista da Universidade de Coimbra* 38 (1999): 335–340.

Foucault, Michel. *Naissance de la Biopolitique, Cours au Collège de France 1978–1979*. Paris: Hautes Etudes, Gallimard-Seuil, 2004.

Fyfe, Paul. "An Archaeology of Victorian Newspapers." *Victorian Periodicals Review* 49, no. 4 (2016): 546–77.

Garnel, Maria Rita. "Médicos e Saúde Pública no Parlamento Republicano." In *Res Publica: cidadania e representação política em Portugal, 1820–1926*, edited by Pedro Almeida, and Fernando Catroga 230–257. Lisbon: Assembleia da República e BNP, 2010.

Garnel, Maria Rita. "Da Régia Escola de Cirurgia à Faculdade de Medicina de Lisboa. O Ensino Médico: 1825–1950." In *A Universidade de Lisboa, séculos XIX-XX*, edited by Sérgio Campos Matos e Jorge Ramos do Ó, Vol. 2, 538–650. Lisbon: Universidade de Lisboa, 2013.

Gougelet, David-Olivier. "The World is One Great Hospital." *Journal of French and Francophone Philosophy* 18 (2008–2010): 43–66.

Graça, Luís. *Diferenciação Socioeconómica dos Praticantes da Arte Médica*. Escola Nacional de Saúde Pública. Accessed 3 June, 2014 http://www.ensp.unl.pt/luis.graca/textos61.html.

Green, Barbara. "Around 1910: Periodical Culture, Women's Writing, and Modernity." *Tulsa Studies in Women's Literature* 30, no. 2 (Fall 2011): 429–439.

Hacking, Ian. *The Taming of Chance*. Cambridge: Cambridge University Press, 1990.

Herman, Edward S., and Noam Chomsky. *Manufacturing Consent. The Political Economy of the Mass Media*. New York: Pantheon Books, 1988.

Hilgartner, Stephen. "The Dominant View of Popularization: Conceptual Problems, Political Uses." *Social Studies of Science* 20 (1990): 519–539.

Jorge, Ricardo. "[Printed letter addressed to the journal]." *MC* 2 (1884): 129.

Judt, Tony. *When the Facts Change. Essays 1995–2010*. Edited by Jennifer Homans. London: William Heinnemann, 2015.

Lathan, Sean. "Affordance and Emergence: Magazine as New Media." *Journal of Victorian Culture Online*. Accessed 3 May, 2016. http://blogs.tandf.co.uk/jvc/2012/12/24/what-is-a-journal-mla2013/.

Lathan, Sean. "The Mess and Muddle of Modernism: The Modernist Journals Project and Modern Periodical Studies." *Tulsa Studies in Women's Literature* 30, no. 2 (Fall 2011): 407–428.

Lathan, Sean, and Robert Sholes. "The Rise of Periodical Studies." *PMLA (journal of the Modern Language Association of America* 121, no. 2 (2006): 517–531.

Lears, T. J. Jackson. "The Concept of Cultural Hegemony: Problems and Possibilities." *The American Historical Review* 90 (1985): 567–9.

Leys, Ruth. "The Turn to Affect: A Critique." *Critical Inquiry* 37 (Spring 2011): 434–463.

Lippmann, Walter. *Public Opinion*. New York: Harcourt, Brace and Company, 1922.

Lippmann, Walter. *The Phantom Public. A Sequel to 'Public Opinion.'*. New York: The MacMillan Company, 1930.

Luz, José Brandão da. "Miguel Bombarda: um materialismo radical." In *História do Pensamento Filosófico Português, O Século XIX*, edited by Pedro Calafate, and Manuel Cândido Pimentel, Vol. 4, 322–349. Lisbon: Editorial Caminho, 2004.

Luz, José Brandão da. "A Propagação do Positivismo." In *vol. 4 of História do Pensamento Filosófico Português. O século XIX*, edited by Pedro Calafate, and Manuel Cândido Pimentel, Vol. 4, 239–432. Lisbon: Editorial Caminho, 2004.

Madureira, Nuno. "A Estatística do Corpo: Antropologia Física e Antropometria na Alvorada do Século XX." *Etnográfica* 2 (2003): 283–303.

Marques, A.H. Oliveira. *História de Portugal 7th ed., 2 vols*. Lisbon: Palas Editores, 1977.

Mergoupi-Savaidou, Eirini, Faidra Papanelopoulou, and Ana Carneiro. ""Popularization of Science and Technology in the "Periphery" A Step Further?" *Technology and Culture* 57 (2016): 966–977.

Michaels, Paula A. "Medical Propaganda and Cultural Revolution in Soviet Kazakhstan, 1918–1941." *The Russian Review* 59 (2000): 159–178.

Miller, Carolyn R. "Genre as Social Action." *Quarterly Journal of Speech* 70 (1984): 151–167.

Mira, Matias Ferreira de. *Manuel Bento de Sousa*. Lisbon: Seara Nova, 1940.

Monteiro, J. M. M. "A Medicina Contemporânea – Um Caso Emblemático na Imprensa Médica Portuguesa." *Unpublished MA dissertation*, Faculdade de Ciências Sociais e Humanas da Universidade Nova de Lisboa, 2012.

Murphy, J. Stephen. "Visualizing Periodical Networks." *The Journal of Modern Periodical Studies* 5, no. 1 (2014): III–XV.

Mussell, James. "The Matter with Media." Accessed 17 June, 2016. https://seeeps.princeton.edu/files/2015/03/mla2013_mussell.pdf.

N.A. "Folhetim: A Syphilis, Tradução do Poema Latino de Fracastor, Livro I." *MC* 1 (1883): 1.

N. A. "Um Principe Médico." *MC* 2 (1884): 31.

N. A. *Association Internationale de la Presse Médicale. Annuaire Générale*. Paris: AIPM, 1906.

Nieto-Galan, Agustí. "Antonio Gramsci Revisited: Historians of Science, Intellectuals, and the Struggle for Hegemony." *History of Science* 49 (2011): 453–478.

Pais, José. *Sousa Martins e suas Memórias Sociais. Sociologia de uma Crença Popular*. Lisboa: Gradiva, 1994.

Papanelopoulou, Faidra, Perdiguero Nieto-Galan Agustí, and Enrique Perdiguero-Gil, eds. *Popularizing Science and Technology in the European Periphery, 1800–2000*. Aldershot: Ashgate, 2009.

Paul, Harry. *The Sorcerer's Apprentice: The French Scientist's Image of German Sciences, 1840–1919*. Gainesville: University of Florida Press, 1972.

Paulo, Zeferino. *Periódicos Portugueses de Medicina e Ciências Subsidiárias*. Lisboa: Instituto para a Alta Cultura, 1944.

Pereira, Ana Leonor. *Darwin em Portugal [1865–1914]. Filosofia. História. Engenharia Social*. Coimbra: Almedina, 2001.

Pereira, José M. "A Evolução da Cultura Médica. A Revista de Neurologia e Psiquiatria (1888–1889)." *Estudos do Século* XX, no. 8 (2008): 365–368.

Pereira, Ana Leonor, and João Rui Pita, eds. *Miguel Bombarda e as Singularidades de uma Época*. Coimbra: Imprensa da Universidade de Coimbra, 2006.

Philpotts, Matthew. "Defining the Thick Journal: Periodical Codes and Common Habitus." 1–5. Accessed 10 November, 2015. https://seeeps.princeton.edu/wpcontent/uploads/sites/243/2015/03/mla2013_philpotts.pdf.

Porter, Roy, ed. *The Popularization of Medicine, 1650–1850*. London: Routledge, 1992.

[Presumably Bombarda]. *MC* 2 (1884): 121.

[Presumably Bombarda]. "As Eleições de Lisboa." *MC* 13, no. 2 (1910): 281–282.

Quental, Antero de. *Causas da Decadência dos Povos Peninsulares nos Últimos Três Séculos (1871)*. Lisbon: Tinta da China, 2008.

Ramos, Rui. "A Formação da *Intelligentsia* Portuguesa (1860–1880)." *Análise Social* 27 (1992): 483–528.

Raposo, Pedro Bettencourt. "Hospitaes: Reflexões sobre o Regime Clínico do Hospital de S. José e Anexos." *MC* 1 (1883): 40–42.

Reis, Carlos V. *História da Ordem dos Médicos – Passado e presente, 2 vols*. Lisbon: CELOM, 2007.

Reis, Fernando Egídio. "Scientific Dissemination in Portuguese Encyclopaedic Periodicals, 1779–1820." *History of Science* 14 (2007): 83–118.

Remoortel, Marianne van. "Joining Forces: European Preirodicals Studies as a New Research Field." *Journal of European Periodical Studies* 1, no. 1 (Summer 2016): 1–3.

Sassoon, Anne S. "The People, Intellectuals and Specialized Knowledge." *Boundary* 2 (1986): 137–68.

Senna, António. *Os Alienados em Portugal*. Lisbon: Publicação de Medicina Contemporânea, 1884–1885, 2 vols.

Shouse, Eric. ""Feeling, Emotion, Affect."." *Journal of Media and Culture*. Accessed 8 January, 2016. http://journal.media-culture.org.au/0512/03-shouse.php.

Silva, Amado J. J., et al. "Miguel Bombarda." *MC* 13 (1910): 321–330.

Simões, Ana, Ana Carneiro, and Maria Paula Diogo. "Riding the Wave to Reach the Masses: Natural Events in Early Twentieth-century Portuguese Daily Press." *Science & Education* 21 (2012): 311–333.

Sousa, Manuel Bento. "A Parvónia." *Lisbon: Typographia de Manuel Jesus Coelho* (1868.

Sousa, José. *O Pensamento Jornalístico Português: Das Origens a Abril de 1974, Vol.1*. Covilhã: LabCom Books, 2010. http://www.labcom-ifp.ubi.pt/book/12.

Steel, John, and Marcel Broersma. "Redefining Journalism during the Period of the Mass Press 1880–1920." *Media History* 21 (2015): 235–237.

Tengarrinha, José. *História da Imprensa Periódica Portuguesa*. Lisbon: Editorial Caminho, 1989.

Topham, Jonathan. "Historicizing 'Popular Science'." *Isis* 100 (2009): 310–318.

[Untitled and unsigned editorial note]. *MC* 2 (1884), 1–2; 49–50; 73–74; 121.

[Untitled and unsigned editorial notes]. *MC* 1 (1883), 1–2; 147–150.

V. AA. "Conselho Superior d'Instrução Pública. Relatorios dos Delegados das Escolas Médicas de Lisboa e Porto." *MC* 5 (1885): 317–318. ; 325–328; 333–340; 342–344; 344–347.

Vieira, Ismael. *Conhecer, tratar e combater a 'peste branca.' A tisiologia e a luta contra a tuberculose em Portugal (1853–1975)*. Porto: CITCEM, 2015.

Weisz, George. "The Emergence of Medical Specialization in the Nineteenth Century." *Bulletin of History of Medicine* 77 (2003): 536–575.

READING PHOTOGRAPHY IN FRENCH NINETEENTH CENTURY JOURNALS

Beatriz Pichel ⓘ

This article explores how photographs published in the French medical and, to some extent, the popular press helped readers to interpret expressions and gestures as signs of emotional states, morbid conditions and physiological and psychological processes. The first two sections examine the use of photography to visualise normal and pathological bodies through measurements and experiments in the medical press, particularly Nouvelle Iconographie de la Salpê-trière, Archives de Neurologie and L'Année Psychologique. The next two sections study how the development of new photographic processes such as the magnesium flash and chrono-photography created new conditions in which the body could be visually scrutinised in the medical press as well as popular journals such as Le Théâtre and the general scientific journal La Nature. This analys results in two main findings: 1) medical journals used photography to assert their own disciplinary identities, and 2) photography acted as a potential bridge between audiences, as some medical and popular journals shared the same beliefs regarding photography's ability to represent the human body, but approached photographic innovations from different, albeit complementary, ways.

Reading the body has always been a key issue in Western medicine, and it became a particularly important skill by the end of the nineteenth century in France.[1] The physiognomic tradition, which associated facial traits to personal characteristics, entered a new phase with the studies on the correlation between facial expressions and emotional states carried out by Duchenne de Boulogne and Darwin in the 1860s and 1870s.[2] During the same years, Alphonse Bertillon applied similar principles to his work at the Police Prefecture in Paris, creating identification systems through the examination of the morphology of the face and other singular marks and the use of photographic portraits.[3] Finally, Jean–Martin Charcot and his team at the Parisian hospital La Salpêtrière developed the anatomo-clinical method based on the visual observation of the body, linking visible symptoms with anatomical and neurological lesions.[4] The bodily language of Charcot's hysterical patients even penetrated into the public sphere as actresses copied some of their most famous gestures.[5] In fin-de-siècle France, the body on display became a means to accessing the emotional, psychological and pathological internal processes that scientists and the public aimed to understand.

This article focuses on two factors that contributed to the shaping and development of this discussion in the late nineteenth century. Firstly, the multiplication of scientific journals and contributors had turned the medical press into a key site where theories were tested, discussed and (eventually) consolidated.[6] Secondly, photography had become a powerful tool in science. Although the objectivity of its images was always challenged, the ability of photography to freeze the subject and to reproduce the images in multiple formats proved very useful in medical and popular contexts.[7] As Geoffrey Belknap has demonstrated, both factors were intertwined.[8] Photographs in the press were not mere illustrations, but had an impact on how science was communicated and understood. Equally, photographs became specific scientific objects when they were published and discussed in journals.[9]

In the following pages, I explore how photographs published in the medical and, to some extent, the popular press helped readers to interpret expressions and gestures as signs of emotional states, morbid conditions and physiological and psychological processes. The first two sections examine the use of photography to visualise normal and pathological bodies through measurements and experiments in the medical press, particularly *Nouvelle Iconographie de la Salpêtrière* (1888–1918, *Nouvelle* hereafter), *Archives de Neurologie* (1870–1907, *Archives* hereafter) and *L'Année Psychologique* (1895 to the present day, *L'Année* hereafter). The next two sections move from the analysis of images to the analysis of technologies, examining how the development of new photographic processes such as the magnesium flash and chronophotography created new conditions in which the body could be visually scrutinised. Taking up Belknap's analysis, these sections consider photography as both a visual tool and a topic of discussion in the medical press as well as popular journals such as *Le Théâtre* (1898–1912) and the general scientific journal *La Nature* (1873–1960).[10]

This investigation applies the concepts and methods of photographic history to the history of the medical press, resulting in two main findings.[11] Firstly, medical journals used photography to assert their own disciplinary identities. As the next sections show, different approaches to psychology and physiology materialised in journals which granted different roles to photography. Secondly, photography acted as a potential bridge between audiences, as some medical and popular journals shared the same beliefs regarding photography's ability to represent the human body, but approached photographic innovations such as artificial lighting from different, albeit complementary ways. In conclusion, tracing photography in medical journals contributes to a better understanding of the medical press as a written visual media, and offers elements of analysis for the study of how related disciplinary fields developed their own identities.

Visualising Bodily Measurements

The first issue of *Nouvelle* opened with a description of its aims. In the spirit of its predecessor *Iconographie photographique de la Salpêtrière* (1875–1880), *Nouvelle* intended to 'make use of the numerous figurative documents that accumulate daily in the Salpêtrière's albums.'[12] The foreword emphasised the value of visual documents, affirming that they 'complete the written observation, bring old cases back to life and facilitate the comparison of analogue cases even when the patient is no longer here.'[13] It continued, 'furthermore, this publication will allow those interested in neurological disorders to judge for themselves.'[14] Photography, therefore, was important not just because it gave 'exact representations' of patients.[15] Doctors at the clinic of nervous diseases at the Salpêtrière valued the taking of the images as much as sharing them with others who might find them useful.

Photographs were intended to open conversations between specialists, and medical journals were the best place to achieve this goal.

Nouvelle situated itself in a particular tradition when its foreword mentioned Iconographie and Archives as its predecessors. The three journals had been founded or directed by Charcot and therefore shared an interest in neuropathology. Désiré Magloire Bourneville, a key figure in the creation of Iconographie and doctor and former intern at the Salpêtrière, became editor-in-chief and a prominent contributor to Archives when he joined the Bicêtre hospital in Paris.[16] In his articles, Bourneville incorporated visual evidence, particularly photographs. The content of these images, and especially the role of the photographs in the articles, created a continuity between Iconographie, Archives and Nouvelle. Visualising the body in photographs taken at hospital came to define the discipline's approach to nervous disorders, and this shared visual culture became the identity mark of the three journals.

One of the ways in which photographs became useful tools in the visualisation of nervous disorders was through bodily measurements. The articles on idiocy written by Bourneville for Archives are good examples. The first of them discussed the case of a child affected of 'severe idiocy, dwarfism and infantilism', and included eight images (Figure 1).[17] All of them corresponded to the same patient, who had been photographed every one or two years since his arrival in 1890.[18] The photographs always followed the same conventions: the child was at the centre of the image, standing up against a dark grey background. Next to him, a scale indicated to the viewer, either the doctor or the journal's reader, the height of the patient. The child was clothed, staring at the camera. Only on one occasion, in 1894 and aged 7, did the patient pose touching the scale and smiling.[19]

All the photographs that accompanied Bourneville's articles presented these characteristics, and two articles published in Nouvelle also compared pathological bodies to a scale.[20] The scale, therefore, had a key role in these journals. Firstly, measuring the body through its comparison to scales linked these images to anthropometric studies such as those carried out by Bertillon, which aimed to quantify the body shape.[21] As Christopher Pinney has argued, anthropometry sought to 'transform the presence of unique bodies into what we might think of as somatic prototypes.'[22] In Bourneville's photographs, the scale displayed visually the individuality of the subject at the same time that categorised it as belonging to a particular group; the 'idiots'.[23] Secondly, the scale brought all the photographs together. Regardless of the particular condition that needed to be highlighted, the scale remained stable, facilitating the comparison among the bodies. Moreover, all the images published in Bourneville's articles were of the same size, and occupied the same place in the page, which reinforced their continuity not only between the photographs belonging to the same article, but between articles over time. The role of the photographs in the articles also remained the same. Photographic images were part of clinical histories, which systematically described the development of the children's bodies and their conditions. The photographs expressed by visual means the same content that was described in the texts.[24] A key element of this repetition was the scale, which provided visual evidence of the figures discussed in the main text.

The visual measurement of the body by means of the standardisation of photographic images became a convention in Archives and Nouvelle, and contributed to the consideration of these photographs as authoritative medical objects. However, other

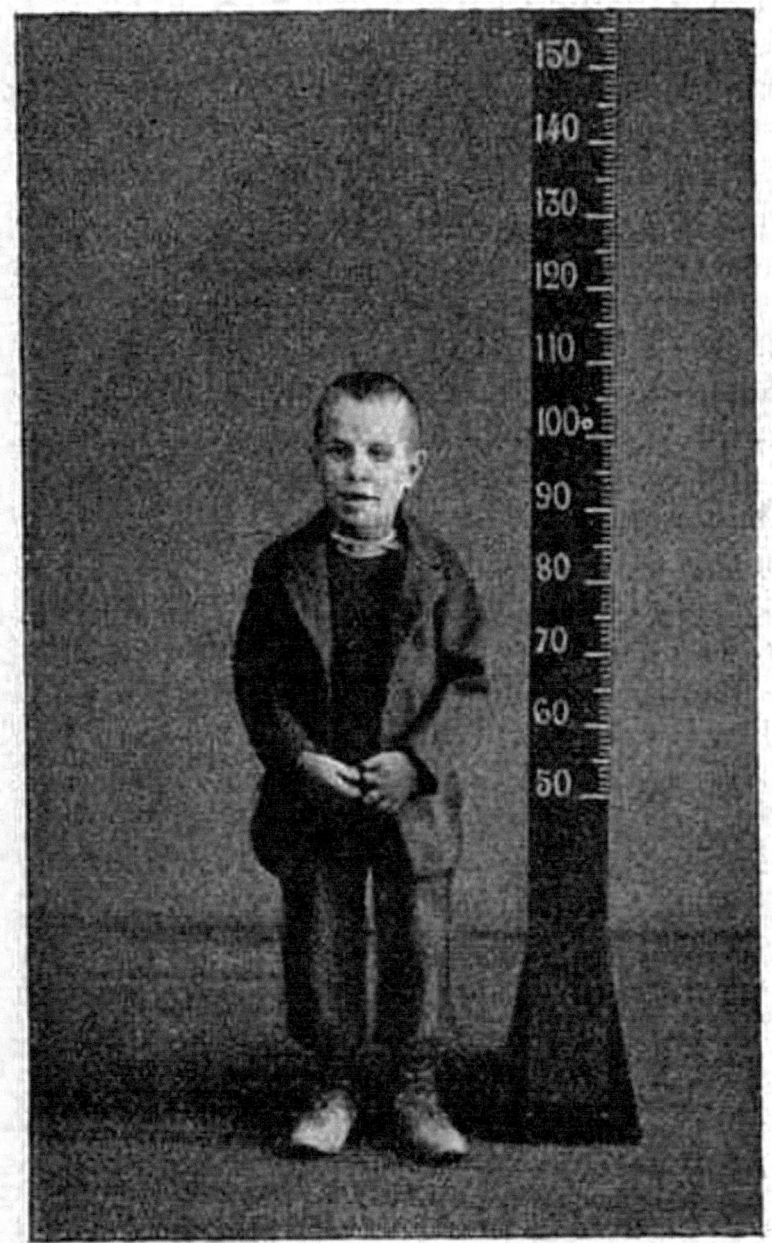

Fig. 7. — Lem..., (Georges) en octobre 1895.

FIGURE 1.
'Lem ... (Georges) en Octobre 1895', Archives de Neurologie, 16 No. 91 (1903), Jubilotheque

disciplines followed different strategies. In 1901, *L'Année* published psychologist Alfred Binet's research on the relation between the measurements of the head and the intelligence of children aged between 11 and 13.[25] In the article, Binet included tables, statistics and one photograph: a portrait of a group of fourteen students at a school in Seine-et-Marne (Figure 2).[26] Seven were sitting on a bench, with their hands on their knees, while the rest stood behind them. They were all wearing school clothes, and stared fixedly at the camera. The wall behind the children suggests that the photograph had been taken outdoors. The fourteen children had been selected out of one hundred due to the different measurements of their heads. Half of them had been classified as 'intelligent', while the other half had been deemed 'unintelligent'. According to Binet,

> By examining these 14 physiognomies, the reader will realise the kind of individual differences that I have found in my subjects. I invite the reader to guess who are, in the group, the most intelligent subjects. This judgement will benefit from the comparison with other physiognomies, while it will encounter more difficulties due to the immobility of the heads and their conventional expression – the living being always more evocative than the photographic portrait.[27]

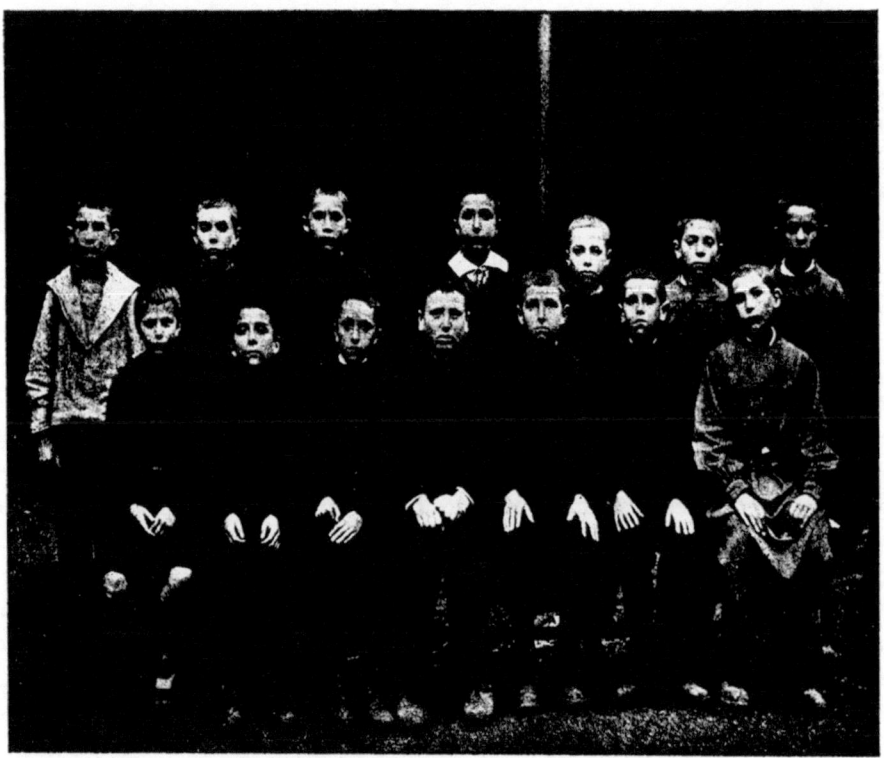

FIo. 1. — Groupe d'enfants d'école primaire, choisis pour la mensuration de la tête.

FIGURE 2.
'Groupe d'enfants d'école primaire, choisis pour la mensuration de la tête', L'anné psychologique, 7 (1901): 357–402. Free of copyright

This paragraph is the only reference to the photograph in the whole article, which went on to discuss calculations on seriation and the average of each of the measurements. In the article, Binet compared numerical figures in tables, which helped to make sense of the correlation between the measurements of the head and the children's intelligence. The photograph, however, compared children to children. The image was not about measurements, but about sizes. The reader could only perceive whose head was bigger, and whose was smaller. This visual exercise was not intended to display the measurements of body parts, but to demonstrate how difficult it was to evaluate the intelligence of children through photographic documents.[28] As the above-mentioned paragraph noted, photographs froze the expression of the children, leaving aside the most interesting nuances of their physiognomy, which contributed to the reader's inability to assess their intelligence. Therefore, while *Archives* presented photographs as a visual aid that reinforced Bourneville's theories, *L'Année* denied that photographs were useful in interpreting bodily measurements.

The visualisation of the children's bodies was nonetheless important. Binet had started his career as an intern in Charcot's service, but he had abandoned the pathological method when he left the Salpêtrière. As head of the Psychology laboratory at the Sorbonne, Binet favoured normal psychology.[29] Accordingly, he photographed children in schools, not in hospitals.[30] Images like Figure 2 mixed intelligent and unintelligent children, stressing the continuity among them. The function of this photograph in the article, therefore, was not to simply visualise the different sizes of children's heads. The publication of such an image in *L'Année* stated the journal's point of view in relation to psychological research. While the photograph did not have specific scientific value (it was not evidence of Binet's theory), it helped to create the identity of the journal and the kind of psychology they supported.

Photography and Medical Experiments

Most of the photographs in *L'Année* were linked to experiments. This is the case for Binet's 'Causerie pédagogique' (1907), which included two photographs of his studies on the breathing of children when they were writing.[31] The images showed the same child in two different postures: the 'ideal attitude', characterised by the straight back and the separation of the chest from the table, and the bad attitude, in which the upper body leaned to the front and to the right, and the table compressed the chest.[32] The reader could also see on the table the child's notebook and Marey's pneumograph, which registered the breathing of the child. The two images, which were included to support the conclusions of the research, were compared to the traces of nasal breathing taken by a pneumograph (visible in the photograph).[33] The graph demonstrated that the position of the child's body did not affect the breathing, contrary to previous research.[34]

The photographs published in *L'Année* were superfluous from a scientific point of view. The images did not play any role in the experiment itself or intervene in the results, but only attested to the fact that the experiment had been performed. These two photographs in particular were misleading, as the compressed chest in the 'bad attitude' photograph might suggest breathing changes. In spite of this, the photographs were important from the point of view of the journal's identity. Firstly, they showed students in a normal environment (not the clinic), focusing again on the normal aspects of psychology. Secondly, they revealed the use of physiological instruments such as Marey's penumograph. Then, the focus of the image was not on the child's body but on the laboratory instrument, which had become a symbol of Binet's experimental psychology.[35]

Contrary to the approach followed by L'Année, other journals attributed a greater role to photography. As Nouvelle's foreword stated, the publication of photographs sought to create a dialogue in the medical community, offering the images for discussion. In the case of experiments, this was particularly important, as photographs made the readers participants in the interpretation of the results. Nouvelle and other journals related to Charcot's school, such as Revue philosophique de la France et l'étranger (1876 to the present day, Revue hereafter) followed this approach. Revue had been founded by Ribot, considered the father of experimental psychology in France, and proponent of the use of the pathological method. It almost never published photographs. As an exception, in 1904 the psychologist and Ribot's mentee Georges Dumas published eight photographs of the experiments he had carried out at the Hôpital de Saint Anne (Figure 3).[36] The experiments, which recalled those originally performed by Duchenne de Boulogne in 1962 and replicated by Charcot and Richer in 1881, consisted of the faradisation of facial muscles and nerves to investigate the pathology of the smile.[37] Dumas, like Duchenne and Charcot before him, photographed the experiments and published the images together with the results.[38] Photographs not only documented the experiments, but played a key role in them. The effects of the faradisation did not last for too long, and were available only to those who observed the experiment. Photography froze the expressions achieved by faradisation, allowing viewers to interpret those expressions, and therefore understanding the role of specific muscles and nerves in producing them. By making these photographs available in the press, the results of the experiment were open for discussion.

Nouvelle and Revue, therefore, integrated photographs into their arguments because they believed readers could interpret visual evidence for their own purposes. Once again, visualising the body was key in these journals. In contrast to this, photographs only served to represent the material settings and instruments in L'Année, whose articles relied on the data provided by tables and graphs.

The Use of Artificial Lighting

Reading the signs of the body was not only a concern in medical journals. The popular press, and in particular the journals specialising in theatre, also sought to provide readers the means to interpret the inner life of the people portrayed in them.[39] Le Théâtre, launched in 1898, intended to make readers feel as if they had attended theatrical representations in Paris and beyond. To achieve this aim, the journal sought to represent with accuracy the artists' performances, and the best means to capture a 'history of gestures' in 'faithful plates' was photography, as journalist Francisque Sarcey argued in the first issue.[40] In this regard, Le Théâtre shared with scientific journals such as Nouvelle the belief that photography's power to freeze the subject in an image would make their expressions readable.

Photographing actors onstage had remained a challenge until the development of the magnesium flash in the late 1880s.[41] While artificial lighting was not standardised

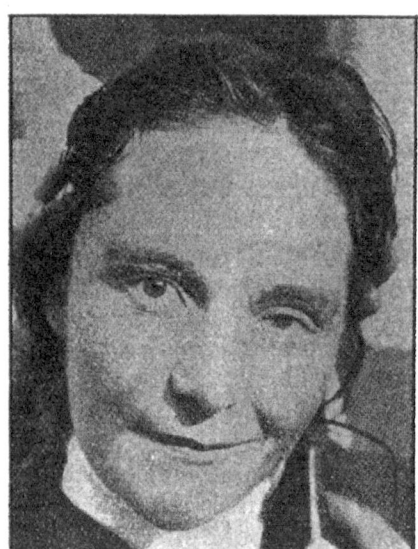

Fig. 59

tions plus simples que nous voulions produire ; nous avons dû chercher des sujets capables de supporter avec impassibilité l'excitation électrique.

Même chez ceux-là, l'expérimentation ne va pas sans difficulté ; trop légère, l'excitation ne produit rien ou ne produit que des contractions trop faibles pour être photographiées ; trop forte, elle provoque des contractions dans tous les muscles du visage. Nous avons dû, avec chaque sujet, tâtonner longtemps pour trouver l'excitation légère qui ne provoque des contractions apparentes que dans les muscles du sourire. Enfin, nous avons choisi de préférence des femmes, pour éviter les inconvénients de la barbe et des moustaches, et nous avons à peine besoin de dire qu'aucun de nos sujets n'a jamais su quelle expression nous cherchions à réaliser ni même que nous cherchions à en réaliser une.

La première photographie est celle de Marie (fig. 59 et 60), la circulaire dont j'ai parlé plus haut, prise dans une période de calme relatif où elle se prêtait volontiers à nos expériences ; la contraction du zygomatique, de l'orbiculaire des paupières et même des releveurs de la lèvre supérieure y est très visible. L'expres-

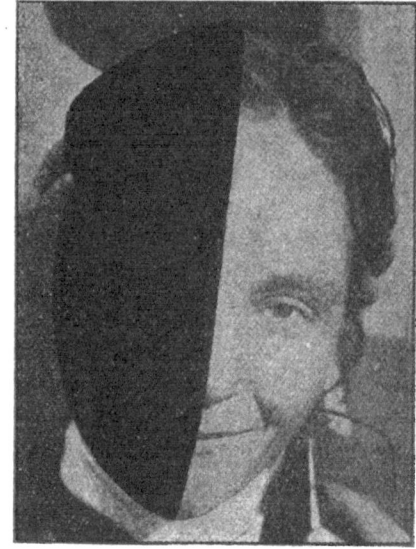

Fig. 60

FIGURE 3.
'Figure 6- Marie' Le sourire, Georges Dumas. Reprinted in Dumas, La Vie Affective. Physiologie - Psychologie - Socialisation (Paris: Presses Universitaires de France, 1948), 208.

until the 1920s, some photographers achieved great success applying flash photography to theatre in the 1890s. One of them was Paul Boyer, from the Van Bosch studios in Paris. In 1892, Boyer had officially introduced his magnesium lamp to the Société Française de la Photographie, although he had been working on it for some years.[42] Unlike the instantaneous flash, which produced a sudden bright light, Boyer's lamp presented two main advantages. Firstly, it produced a continuous source of light, which allowed actors to get used to the light before the shutter was released. Secondly, several lamps could be linked to each other, so the light covered large stages.[43] Boyer's innovative photographs of the plays represented in the main Parisian theatres were described in newspapers such as *Le Figaro*, *Le Petit Parisienne* and *Le Journal*, and were published in *Le Photo-Programme* between 1895 and 1896. Boyer was also the photographer of most of the photographs in *Le Théâtre*, which proudly announced in its first number that readers would be able not only to see his 'artworks', but also to order enlargements of their favourite images. [44]

While the popular press showed Boyer's photographs and praised its quality, it did not comment on the problems involved in photographing actors, or on the qualities of the magnesium flash. This discussion happened in specialised journals such as the *Bulletin de la Société Française de la Photographie* and *Photo-Gazette*, targeted at professional photographers, as well as in scientific publications. *La Nature*, a popular science periodical founded by Gaston Tissandier, often disseminated the latest photographic procedures, such as colour and instantaneous photography.[45] In 1888, some years before Boyer's magnesium lamp, it had published G Mareschal's 'Photography in the theatre', which explained how the photographer M Balagny had successfully captured live photographs of the representation of *Chatte Blanche* at the Châtelet theatre in Paris. In this case, two factors had come together: the availability of electrical lighting in the theatre, and Balagny's production of soft plaques and inextensible films (Figure 4).[46] Balagny's method was different from Boyer's, as he took advantage of the electrical lighting of the room, while Boyer and others worked on improving the use of artificial bright light that directly illuminated the subject. The innovations in this field were duly reported by *La Nature*, which took a great interest in the scientific explanations of artificial lighting.[47]

Mareschal's article in *La Nature* included one of the six images that Balagny had taken at the Châtelet theatre. As usual in this journal, the photograph was reproduced as a facsimile of an engraving. As Belknap has argued, the fact that the image was consumed by the public as an engraving did not dismiss its authority, as it had been reproduced from a photograph.[48] The bottom of the image allows us to see the stage's footlights, which gave an indication of the technology used to illuminate the stage and therefore to produce the photograph. The engraving fulfilled the aims of the article. However, the quality of the reproduction prevented the reader from checking whether the photograph had captured the actors' performance with enough detail. If readers wanted to see the actors' gestures, they had to turn to *Le Théâtre*, *L'Illustration théâtrale* or *Le Photo-Programme*.

Popular and scientific journals tackled the application of artificial lighting to photography in the 1890s in different but complementary ways. While the scientific press was more concerned about the technological procedures that made the photography of actors possible, the popular press was interested in the resulting images. These two aspects of the same problem were very rarely addressed in the same space. An exception to this rule is *Photo-Journal*, a specialised photographic journal which combined theatrical reviews, discussions of technical aspects of photography (including artificial lighting) and good quality images, reproduced through the photo-mechanical process.[49] Despite the different approaches to artificial lighting in these journals, they all had a common aim. Capturing the actors' best performances was not only *Le Théâtre*'s goal. Contributors to *La*

LA PHOTOGRAPHIE AU THÉÂTRE

Nous avons parlé souvent des photographies instantanées, et nos lecteurs ont eu sous les yeux des spécimens de ce qu'on peut obtenir dans ce genre par les procédés actuels; mais, jusqu'à présent on s'est borné à faire des épreuves en plein air et au soleil. Nous avons voulu nous rendre compte du résultat qu'on pouvait obtenir à la lumière artificielle et pour cela nous nous sommes adressés à M. Balagny, l'inventeur des plaques souples et des papiers pelliculaires inextensibles fabriqués par MM. Lu

mière. Nous avions déjà eu l'occasion, dans des expériences précédentes[1], d'apprécier la sensibilité de ces produits et nous avions confiance dans le résultat. Nous ne nous étions pas trompé. L'expérience s'est faite au théâtre du Châtelet, qui est éclairé à la lumière électrique, pendant les représentations de la *Chatte Blanche*; le directeur, M. Floury, avait bien voulu mettre à cet effet une loge à notre disposition et nous sommes heureux de pouvoir l'en remercier ici. M. Balagny est parvenu à faire six clichés (dimensions : 18 sur 24) sur papier pelliculaire, représentant les principaux tableaux de cette féerie. Il ne fallait pas penser au traditionnel « *ne*

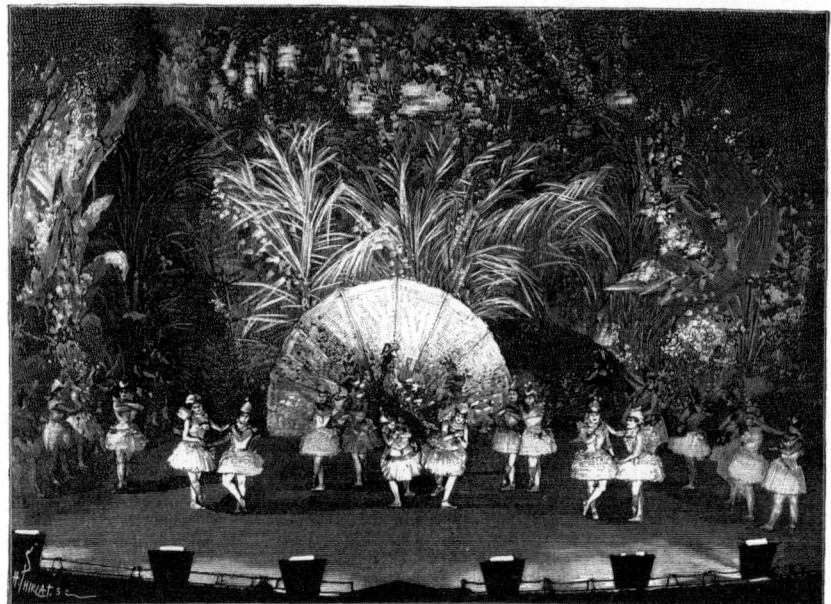

Un ballet de la *Chatte Blanche*, féerie du Théâtre du Châtelet à Paris. — Fac-similé d'une photographie exécutée par M. Balagny, pendant une représentation.

bougeons plus » et, par conséquent, la pose devait être très courte; elle a varié de *un quart* de seconde à *deux* secondes. Le cliché que reproduit la gravure en fac-similé qui accompagne cet article a été obtenu en *moins d'une* seconde. Disons un mot des procédés employés :

Les *plaques souples* sont formées d'une feuille de gélatine transparente qui sert de support à la couche de gélatino-bromure; elles se traitent comme les glaces sur lesquelles elles ont l'avantage de ne pas casser et de peser infiniment moins.

Quant au papier pelliculaire, qui présente les mêmes avantages, il se traite de la même manière; mais, lorsque le cliché est terminé, le papier s'enlève avec la plus grande facilité, et il ne reste plus que

la pellicule avec laquelle on tire directement les épreuves.

La difficulté pour que ces procédés soient pratiques, consistait à rendre la gélatine *inextensible*, de manière à ne pas avoir de déformation du cliché pendant les différentes opérations du développement et du fixage; cette difficulté a été vaincue par M. Balagny, et c'est le secret de fabrication. Le papier paraît être plus sensible encore que la plaque souple et l'inventeur attribue ce résultat à l'opacité du support; dans tous les cas cette opacité empêche l'auréole de se produire autour des points très lumineux, comme cela arrive avec les glaces par suite de la

[1] Voy. n° 755, du 19 novembre 1887, p. 597.

FIGURE 4.
'Un ballet de la Chatte Blanche, féérie du Théâtre du Chatelet à Paris', La Nature, 16, n. 757–782 (1888): 93. Cnum-Conservatoire numérique des Arts et Métiers

Nature also hoped that this new procedure would be able to make good images of theatrical representations, and the photographers writing in *Bulletin* also congratulated Boyer for his work in achieving this aim. While their approaches differed, scientific, popular and photographic journals shared the same concerns regarding the use of photography as a means to understanding the external signs of the body. In this regard, the discussions on artificial lighting and the images of theatrical representations were not very different from the debates in the medical press previously examined. In fact, Albert Londe, Head of the photographic service at the Salpêtrière and photographer of most of the photographs published in *Nouvelle*, also used the magnesium flash in his work.[50] Together with photographic measurements and experiments, artificial lighting became a discussion point in the quest to determine the best methods for reading normal and pathological bodies.

The Case for Chronophotography

Besides artificial lighting, the other photographic technology widely discussed in the French press was instantaneous photography, and particularly chronophotography. First invented by Eadweard Muybridge in 1877, chronophotography was the taking of several instantaneous images at regular (short) intervals of time to capture a subject in movement.[51] The discussion of this new photographic application in the press shaped the terms of the debate.[52] While it was mainly the medical and scientific press that engaged with this conversation, the ability to capture movement soon attracted the performing arts. Around 1893, Londe took several chronophotographs intended to help artists to represent nature and the human body in an accurate way. Among these images, Londe portrayed an acrobat kneeling on the trapeze.[53] These chronophotographic images are very similar in their content to the photographs Londe took at the Parisian Hippodrome de l'Alma in the late 1880s, and later in 1891 as part of his experiments with artificial lighting.[54] Londe was not the only one who applied chronophotography to capture performances. Georges Demenÿ, assistant of Marey at the Station Physiologique, also photographed 'the cry and gesture of a famous actor' in the context of his experiments on chronophotography.[55] This series recalled Demenÿ's famous 'living portraits', chronophotographic close-ups that showed in details the facial muscles involved in different utterances, such as 'je t'aime' and 'vive la France'.[56] Both Demenÿ's and Londe's projects linked the improvement of photographic technologies with a better or more accurate visual representation of the human body in movement. In this regard, the conversation around chronophotography was similar to the discussions on artificial lighting previously examined. As the following will show, both Demenÿ's and Londe's chronophotographic methods were also used in the medical press to strengthen approaches to the body in different disciplines, as discussed in the first two sections of this article.

Unsurprisingly, the two medical journals that engaged the most with chronophotography were *Nouvelle* and *L'Année*. In the case of *Nouvelle*, the link with chronophotography was evident. Londe had designed his own chronophotographic camera to help Paul Richer in his research on the physiology of movement, and opened an outdoors studio at the Salpêtrière specially adapted to their needs.[57] In the spirit of sharing the visual documents produced at the Salpêtrière, *Nouvelle* published in 1895 an article by Richer on the shape of the body in movement, fully illustrated with Londe's chronophotographs of a naked man lifting weights.[58] In the same vein, Demenÿ wrote an article for *L'Année* in 1898 featuring Marey's work at the Station Physiologique.[59] In it, Demenÿ explained in detailed the technical characteristics and functioning of his chronophotographic camera, with the aim of insisting 'on the role that [chronophotography] can play in physiology laboratories'.[60]

Both Marey and Londe's chronophotographic methods were intended to enhance visual perception by rendering visible what escaped the human eye. However, the visualisation of movement followed different principles in each case: while Marey intended to measure the direction and speed of movement, Londe wanted to reveal the external changes in the muscles produced by movement.[61] These two purposes required different cameras. Marey constructed a single lens camera that analysed movement by capturing a succession of photographic images, and synthesised it through its filmic projection. The figures were recorded on the same plate, which often produced overlaps. Marey and Demenÿ's approach corresponded to the interests of experimental physiology, as they used chronophotography to translate the visible world into data that would later be analysed.[62]

In contrast, Londe was interested in the external shape of the body. While the direction of the movement was important in cases of pathological locomotion, in the studies of normal physiology the focus was on the visible changes experienced by the muscles. To this end, Londe built a camera with twelve shutters that were shot successively on the same plate.[63] The final image consisted of three rows of four columns, each showing an instant of the movement with no overlapping whatsoever. Unlike Marey, Londe sought to highlight the body of the subject, and photographed the subjects naked against a grey background. Even if Richer's project was on physiology and not pathology, this method followed the principles of the anatomo-clinical medicine. As with the indoor studio Londe had set up at the Salpêtrière, his chronophotographic camera, outdoor stage and plates were designed to enhance the visual observation of the body.

The publication of Demenÿ's article in *L'Année* was the journal's stance on how to use chronophotography. Binet had written a review in 1895 praising Richer's *Physiologie Artistique*, recognising the relevance of the study to psychology.[64] He mentioned the chronophotographs that illustrated the book, but only to recall Marey's and Demenÿ's work, without even mentioning Londe. On the other hand, *Nouvelle* did not show Marey's work, concentrating on Londe's approach to chronophotography. The different ways in which *L'Année* and *Nouvelle* featured this photographic invention provide a good example of how particular photographic technologies identified with the scientific aims and methods of each publication. The only outlet that frequently published works by both authors was *La Nature*, which took a broad approach to science and never identified with a single school of thought. Journals, therefore, became a privileged site not only to discuss the technical details and potential uses of chronophotography, but also the different disciplinary approaches to the visualisation of the body in movement.

Conclusion

The survey of the role of photography in major journals in French psychology and physiology (*Nouvelle*, *Archives* and *L'Année*) and others such as *Le Théâtre* and *La Nature* have demonstrated that photographic reproductions in the press became a key site where ideas regarding the body, its external signs and their interpretation were discussed. Most of the contributors examined in this article defended the accuracy of photographs in representing fleeting expressions, but not all of them. As we have seen, Binet maintained that photographs were not able to convey natural expressions. This disagreement reflected tensions between disciplines and schools of thought, and projected different images of science. While *L'Année* represented psychology as an activity involving physiological experiments and instruments, *Nouvelle*, *Archives* and *Revue* reinforced visual observation through the display of bodily pathologies in the clinic. Both images of science were commented on in *La Nature*, but only one penetrated into popular journals. *Le Théâtre*'s belief that photographs allowed the truthful representation of actors' performances, and that the publication of these images in journals would enable a history of gestures, connected it with the aims and practices of *Nouvelle*.

Photographs printed in the press became objects of a particular kind, different from the prints stored in hospitals and photographic studios. In this move, photographs brought together and drew apart different fields. Medical journals reaffirmed their own disciplinary identities through the role they granted to photographs. But, as Demenÿ's chronophotographs of an actor show, photographs were mixed material that circulated across spaces: the same image could be published in a psychology journal and also contribute to theatre studies. Photographs did not belong to either theatre or science, but was what connected both fields.

Acknowledgment

This research was presented for the first time at the conference "Working with Nineteenth-Century Medicine and Health Periodicals", Saint Anne College, University of Oxford, 16 May 2015. I wanted to thank Sally Frampton and Jennifer Wallis for inviting me to contribute to this Special Issue. I also wanted to thank the two anonymous reviewers for their insightful comments, and the Wellcome Trust for making this article available in Open Access.

Disclosure Statement

No potential conflict of interest was reported by the author.

Funding

This work was supported by the Wellcome Trust [grant number 103101/Z/13/Z].

Notes

1. See Callen, *The Spectacular Body* and Wallis, *Investigating the Body*.
2. Duchenne, *Mécanisme*; Darwin, *The Expression*. See Delaporte, *Anatomie*.
3. Kalunszynski, "Alphonse Bertillon."

4. Goetz, "Jean Martin Charcot," 203–212.

5. Gordon, "From Charcot," Gordon, *Why the French*, also Gilman, "The Image," 345–436; Justice-Mallow, "Charcot," 133–138. See also Didi-Huberman, *Invention of Hysteria*; Hunter, *The Face* and Hustvedt, *Medical Muses*.

6. Belknap, *From a Photograph*, 6. There was also a surge in the popular press, see Gervais, *La Fabrique*.

7. On science and photography, see Tucker, *Nature Exposed*; Wilder, *Photography* and Daston & Galison, *Objectivity*.

8. Belknap, *From a Photograph*.

9. Elizabeth Edwards has argued that the materiality of the photographic prints contributed to their consideration as scientific objects in "Material Beings," 71.

10. Belknap, *From a Photograph*, 6.

11. Ibid.; Edwards and Hart, *Photographs, Objects, Histories*.

12. Richer, Tourette, and Londe, "Avertissement."

13. Ibid.

14. Ibid.

15. Ibid.

16. Faure, "La photographie," 104–124.

17. Bourneville, "Idiotie profonde," 38–55.

18. The text mentions the years 1890, 1892, 1894, 1895, 1896, 1897, 1899 and 1902. Ibid., 41, 43, 44, 45, 47, 48, 49 and 51.

19. Ibid., 44.

20. See for instance the series of articles on a patient suffering from idiocy and myxomatosis who had recently died. Bourneville, "Fin de l'histoire," 97–119.

21. Brown, "Racialising the Virile Body," 631.

22. Pinney, *Photography and Anthropology*, 29. See also Brown, "Racialising the Virile Body."

23. Bourneville, "Idiotie profonde," 38–55.

24. Something similar happened in the examples examined by Mark Jackson in "Images of Deviance," 319–337.

25. On the history of *L'Année*, see Vermès, "L'Année Psychologique," 113–129.

26. Binet, "Recherches complémentaires," 375–402.

27. Ibid, 382.

28. Ibid, 382.

29. See Plas, "Psychology," 91–107, Nicolas and Charvillat, "Introducing Psychology," 143–164, and Nicolas, Segui and Lefrand, "Les premières revues," 71–110.

30. Binet's relationship with images has been examined by Mireille Berton, "Alfred Binet," 197–202.

31. Binet, "Causerie pédagogique," 405–431.

32. Ibid., 428.

33. Ibid. 428

34. Binet cited here the work of Dr Badaloni, who had demonstrated a correlation between bad posture, where the table compresses the chest of the child, and the decrease of breathing. Ibid. 425–428.

35. Evans, "Psychological Instruments," 113–129.

36. Dumas, "Le sourire," 1–23.

37. Duchenne (de Boulogne), *Mécanisme*, Charcot and Richer "Contribution," 32–75.
38. I have discussed these photographs in Pichel, "Die Psychologie."
39. The next two sections will focus on photography, but similar analyses have been carried out by Mireille Berton in relation to cinema and psychology (Berton, *Le Corps*) and by Garcin Marrou regarding theatre and psychology (Garcin Marrou, "André de Lorde").
40. Sarcey, "Le théâtre instantané"
41. While the first experiments with magnesium started in the 1860s with Alfred Brothers and Charles Piazzi, the magnesium flash powders were not introduced until the late 1880s. Pritchard, "Artificial Lighting." For a cultural history of flash, see Kate Flint, *Flash!*.
42. S.G.D.G., "Lampe-éclaire Boyer," 160–162.
43. Ibid., 160.
44. *Le Théâtre*, n. 1, January 1898.
45. On *La Nature*, see Manuel Chemineau, *Fortunes*.
46. Mareschal, "La Photographie", 93.
47. for instance Londe, "Photographie instantanée," 343–346.
48. Belknap, *From a Photograph*.
49. Peutat, "Derrière le Rideau," 97–99.
50. Londe, "Contribution à l'étude," 102–103.
51. On Muybridge, see Braun, *Muybridge*.
52. Belknap, *From a Photograph*, 152.
53. Londe, *Album de chronophotographies*, plate XV.
54. Londe's photographs of acrobats at the Hippodrome de l'alma are available online at the Musée d'Orsay, "Album composé dans l'entourage d'Albert Londe" http://www.musee-orsay.fr/en/collections/index-of-works/notice.html?no_cache=1&ens=1&nnumid=172164&retouroeuvre=%252Fen%252Fcollections%252Findex-of-works%252Fnotice.html%253Fno_cache%253D1%2526zsz%253D5%2526lnum%253D8. Accessed on February 1, 2018.
55. Demenÿ, "Les appareils chronophotographiques," 367.
56. Demenÿ, "Le portrait," 1–4.
57. Londe, "La photochronographie," 370–374.
58. Richer, "De la forme," 122–135.
59. Demenÿ, "Les appareils chronophotographiques," 347–368.
60. Ibid., 368.
61. See Braun and Whitcombe, "Marey, Muybridge," 218.
62. Braun, *Picturing Time*.
63. Londe, "La photochronographie," 370–374.
64. Binet, "P. Richer," 731–740.

ORCID

Beatriz Pichel ⓘ http://orcid.org/0000-0002-7542-2852

Bibliography

Belknap, Geoffrey. *From a Photograph. Authenticity, Science and the Periodical Press 1870–1890*. London: Bloomsbury, 2016.

Berton, Mireille. "Alfred Binet, entre illusionnisme, spiritisme et cinéma des origins." *Recherches & Educations* 1 (2008): 197–202.

Berton, Mireille. *Le Corps nerveux des spectateurs. Cinéma et sciences du psychisme autour de 1900.* Lausanne: L'Âge d'Homme, 2015.

Binet, Alfred. "P. Richer. Physiologie Artistique." *L'Année Psychologique* 2 (1895): 731–740.

Binet, Alfred. "Recherches complémentaires de céphalométrie sur 100 enfants d'intelligence inégale, choisis dans les écoles primaires du département de Seine-et-Marne." *L'Année Psychologique* 7 (1900): 375–402.

Binet, Alfred. "Causerie pédagogique." *L'Année Psychologique* 14 (1907): 405–431.

Bourneville, Désiré. "Fin de l'histoire d'un idiot myxœdématuex." *Archives de Neurologie* 16, no. 92 (1903): 97–119.

Bourneville, Désiré. "Idiotie profonde avec nanisme et infantilisme. Amélioration considerable." *Archives de Neurologie* 16, no. 91 (1903): 38–55.

Braun, Marta. *Picturing Time. The Work of Étienne-Jules Marey (1830–1904).* Chicago: University of Chicago Press, 1992.

Braun, Marta. *Eadweard Muybridge.* London: Reaktion Books, 2010.

Braun, Marta, and Elizabeth Whitcombe. "Marey, Muybridge, and Londe: The Photography of Pathological Locomotion." *History of Photography* 23, no. 3 (1999): 218–224.

Brown, Elspeth. "Racialising the Virile Body: Eadweard Muybridge's Locomotion Studies 1883–1887." *Gender & History* 17, no. 3 (2011): 627–656.

Callen, Anthea. *The Spectacular Body. Science, Method and Meaning in the Work of Degas.* New Haven; London: Yale University Press, 1995.

Charcot, Jean-Martin, and Paul Richer. 1882. "Contribution a l'étude de l'hypnotisme chez les hystériques. Du phenomène de l'hyperexcitabilité neuromusculaire." *Archives de neurologie* III: 310–319.

Chemineau, Manuel. *Fortunes de la Nature, 1873–1914.* Berlin: LIT Verlag, 2012.

Darwin, Charles. *The Expression of Emotions in Man and Animals.* London: John Murray, 1872.

Daston, Lorraine, and Peter Galison. *Objectivity.* New York: Zone Books, 2007.

Delaporte, François. *Anatomie des Passions.* Paris: PUF, 2003.

Demenÿ, Georges. *Le portrait vivant.* Paris: Impr. de L. Dechristépère, 1892.

Demenÿ, Georges. "Les appareils chronophotographiques." *L'Année Psychologique* 5 (1898): 347–386.

Didi-Huberman, Georges. *Invention of Hysteria. Charcot and the Photographic Iconography at the Salpêtrière.* Translated by Alisa Hartz. Cambridge, MA: The MIT Press, 2003.

Duchenne (de Boulogne), Benjamin Guillaume. *Mécanisme de la physionomie humaine, ou analyse électro-physiologique de l'expression des passions.* Paris: Jules Renouard, 1862.

Dumas, Georges. "Le Sourire. Étude psycho-physiologique." *Revue philosophique de la France et l'étranger* 7 (1904): 1–23.

Edwards, Elizabeth. "Material Beings: Objecthood and Ethnographic Photographs." *Visual Studies* 17, no. 1 (2002): 67–75.

Edwards, Elizabeth, and Janice Hart. *Photographs, Objects, History. On the Materiality of Images.* London: Routledge, 2004.

Evans, Rand B. "Psychological Instruments at the Turn of the Century." *American Psychologist* 55, no. 3 (2000): 113–129.

Faure, Marie-Rose. "La photographie scientifique de Bourneville." *Communication et langages* 135 (2003): 104–124.

Flint, Kate. *Flash! Photography, Writing and Surprising Illumination*. Oxford: Oxford University Press, 2017.

Garcin Marrou, Flore. 2011. "André de Lorde et Alfred Binet: quand le théâtre du Grand-Guignol passionne les scientifiques." *Recherches & Educations* 5: 193–204.

Gervais, Thierry. *La fabrique de l'information visuelle. Photographies et magazines d'actualité*. Paris: Textuel, 2015.

Gilman, Sander. "The Image of the Hysteric." In *Hysteria Beyond Freud*, edited by Sander Gilman, Helen King, Roy Porter, and Eleine Showalter, 345–436. Berkeley: University of California Press, 1993.

Goetz, Christopher G. "Jean-Martin Charcot and the Anatomo-Clinical Method of Neurology." *Handbook of Clinical Neurology* 95 (2009): 203–212.

Gordon, Rae Beth. *Why the French Love Jerry Lewis. From Cabaret to Early Cinema*. Standford: Standford University Press, 2001.

Gordon, Rae Beth. "From Charcot to Charlot: Unconscious Imitation and Spectatorship in French Cabaret and Early Cinema." In *The Mind of Modernism*, edited by Mark S. Micale, 93–124. Stanford, CA: Stanford University Press, 2004.

Hunter, Mary. *The Face of Medicine. Visualising Medical Masculinities in Late Nineteenth Century Paris*. Manchester: Manchester University Press, 2016.

Hustvedt, Asti. *Medical Muses. Hysteria in Nineteenth-Century Paris*. London: Bloomsbury, 2011.

Jackson, Mark. "Images of Deviance: Visual Representations of Mental Defectives in Early Twentieth-Century Medical Texts." *The British Journal for the History of Science* 28, no. 3 (1995): 319–337.

Justice-Mallow, Rhona. "Charcot and the Theatre of Hysteria." *Journal of Popular Culture* 28, no. 4 (1995): 133–138.

Kalunszunski, Martine. "Alphone Bertillon et l'anthropométrie judiciaire. L'identification au coeur de l'ordre républicain." *Criminocorpus*, Online Since 12 May 2014. Consultated on 1 February 2018.

Londe, Albert. 1892. "Contribution à l'étude des lumières artificielles en photographie." *Bulletin de la Société Française de Photographie* tome III, vol 4: 102–103.

Londe, Albert. "La photochronographie dans les sciences médicales. Le nouveau laboratoire de la Salpêtrière." *La Nature* 21 (1893): 370–374.

Londe, Albert. *Album de Chronophotographies Documentaires à l'Usage des Artistes*. Paris: Charles Mendel, 1903.

Londe, Albert. "Photographie instantané et chronophotographie pendant l'éclair magnésique." *La Nature* 31 (1903): 343–346.

Mareshal, G. 1888. "La photographie au théâtre." *La Nature* 16: 93–94.

Nicolas, Serge, and Agnès Charvillat. "Introducing Psychology as an Academic Discipline in France: Théodule Ribot and the Collège de France (1888–1901)." *Journal of the History of Behavioural Sciences* 37, no. 2 (2001): 143–164.

Nicolas, Serge, Juan Segui, and Ludovic Ferrand. "Les premières revues de psychologie. La place de *L'Année Psychologique*." *L'Année Psychologique* 100, no. 1 (2000): 71–110.

Peutat, Georges. "Derrière le rideau." *Photo-journal* (1891): 97–99.

Pichel, Beatriz. "Die Psychologie Des Lächelns Bei Georges Dumas. Eine fotogeschichtliche Studie." *Fotogeschichte* 140, no. 36 (2016): 13–24.

Pinney, Christoper. *Photography and Anthropology*. London: Reaktion Books, 2011.

Plas, Regine. "Psychology and Psychical Research in France Around the End of the Nineteenth Century." *History of the Human Sciences* 25, no. 2 (2012): 91–107.

Pritchard, Michael. "Artificial Lighting." In *Encyclopedia of Nineteenth Century Photography*, edited by John Hanavy, vol. I, 83–84. London: Routledge, 2008.

Richer, Paul. "De la forme du corps en mouvement." *Nouvelle Iconographie de la Salpêtrière* 8 (1895): 122–135.

Richer, Paul, Gilles de la Tourette, and Albert Londe. "Avertissement." *Nouvelle Iconographie de la Salpêtrière* 1 (1888): 1–4.

Sarcey, Francisque. 1898. "Le théâtre instantané." *Le Théâtre* 1: 1.

S.G.D.G. 1892. "Lampe-éclair Boyer." *Bulletin de la Société Française de la Photographie* tome III, vol. 4: 160–162. 5 February.

Tucker, Jennifer. *Nature Exposed. Photography as Eyewitness in Victorian Science*. Baltimore: Johns Hopkins University Press, 2005.

Vermès, Geneviève. "*L'Année Psychologique* et son réseau: lectures et fabrication d'une nouvelle discipline, 1894–1927." *L'Année Psychologique* 96 (1996): 113–129.

Wallis, Jennifer. 2017. *Investigating the Body in the Victorian Asylum. Doctors, Patients, and Practices*. Basingstoke, Hampshire: Palgrave Macmillan.

Wilder, Kelley. *Photography and Science*. London: Reaktion Books, 2009.

'BICYCLE-FACE' AND 'LAWN TENNIS' GIRLS

Debating girls' health in late nineteenth- and early twentieth-century British periodicals

Hilary Marland

In the final quarter of the nineteenth century, as periodical literature itself diversified and increased in volume, a growing amount of copy was devoted to the medical issues of the day, including debates about the limits of young women's energy and the impact of the extension of their activities in education, public life and sport on their health and vitality, and their future role as mothers. The article explores the ways in which doctors in particular utilized these outlets to convey their opinions and concerns, revealing a great diversity of viewpoints as well as the flexible editorial policies of many of these journals. Both male and a growing cohort of female doctors employed the platform of the periodical to popularize and make relevant medical ideas, while also building on, highlighting and creating broader cultural and gendered perspectives and emblems of girlhood.

Research into representations of girls' health and health advice for young women in the late nineteenth and early twentieth centuries has highlighted the extent to which medical, popular health and general interest periodicals and magazines debated girls' capacity for improving their well-being and vitality, particularly in relation to their ambitions to engage in new public, educational and sporting activities.[1] A vast diversity of print media—health advice manuals, pamphlets and tracts, newspapers, magazines as well as journals—discussed girls' potential to enhance their health, and the ways they might achieve this, or, conversely, by pitting their slender physical and mental resources against overlarge challenges, their potential for ruin: 'Troubles ahead for Women'.[2] Editorials, leading articles, health columns and letters pages examined and re-examined the issue of girls' ability to develop their ambitions in secondary and higher education and the benefits of sports and exercise. They also debated the impact that mental and physical exertion might have on young women's developing bodies, minds and capacity for future motherhood, the limits of girls' energy, and the relationship between bodily and mental strain and gain. Such pieces featured, among many other outlets, in major literary and general interest journals, such as *The Nineteenth Century*, *The Fortnightly Review* and *The Saturday Review*, the evangelical family magazine, *The Leisure Hour*, the reform-orientated digest *Review of Reviews* and *The Woman's Signal*, with its focus on temperance reform, feminist issues and women's employment, lay health periodicals, such as *Health* and

Good Health, and a growing number of magazines devoted to women and girl readers. The potential and dangers of new educational, vocational and physical challenges were criticized and contested or advocated and welcomed by an equally broad range of authorities on this topic: medical practitioners, including a growing cohort of women doctors, headmistress and teachers, gymnastics instructors, journalists, social commentators and feminists.

Notably, as Kate Flint has remarked, doctors engaged more extensively with wider publics through their published work from the 1870s onwards, not least on the subject of the relationship between health and female education, as debate on this topic 'spread from specialist texts to a range of publications with the potential to reach a wider readership'.[3] Increasingly too, journalists and other contributors to periodicals cited the published work or opinions of medical men and women, drawing on their sometimes provocative viewpoints to produce topical opinion pieces. These trends were boosted in 1874 following an influential exchange between eminent psychiatrist, Dr Henry Maudsley, best known for his views on social and mental degeneration, and Dr Elizabeth Garrett Anderson, the first Englishwoman to qualify as a physician and surgeon, suffragette and active supporter of higher education for girls, on the relationship between study and the health and reproductive capacity of young women.[4] The debate took place not in a medical journal as we might expect, but in two issues of *The Fortnightly Review*, a wide-circulation periodical renowned for its engagement with the topics of the day, and for publishing articles that dealt with female emancipation and reform in academia and the workplace.

Maudsley warned in his lengthy article, 'Sex in Mind and in Education', that appeared in the April edition of the *The Fortnightly Review*, that overspending vital energy would produce menstrual disorders and mental collapse, and potentially destroy young women's future capacity to bear healthy children.[5] His piece gave credence to a theory that was to dominate the late Victorian era and persist well beyond it, that the body—particularly the female body—contained a limited supply of vital energy to fuel its physical and mental activities, and 'what was spent in one period was bound to be missed in another'.[6] Garrett Anderson's robust rejoinder was published in the following issue of the periodical, and argued that, provided teachers took care to monitor girls' health and protect them from mental fatigue and excessive physical activity, study was unlikely to be a threat to their well-being. Indeed, it was likely to enhance health; headmistresses and other reformers had sought, she avowed, with marked success to improve, through exercise and hygienic practices, the physical development of girls alongside their mental training.[7] This controversy and its repercussions have been covered in detail elsewhere, but its significance lay not just in its impact on deliberations about young women's health in the scientific press, but also for the way it was taken up in articles and discussion pieces in a huge number of outlets, some liberal and reformist, and many not, that continued to appear on this topic in the decades to follow, exemplifying the potential of the periodical as a means of communicating important medical topics and viewpoints.[8]

The Victorian period saw a rapid expansion in the number and range of periodicals, 'a pervasiveness of periodical literature', a process that Vann and VanArsdel have attributed to advances in printing techniques, lower printing costs (and thus lower purchasing prices), and new channels of distribution, but most significantly to the potential for this widely circulated print media to document and contribute to the cultural shift from less sophisti-cated and less urbanized times to the modern era.[9] Significantly, when girls' health was dis-cussed, it was often set in the context of urban growth and a rapidly changing environment, which offered a particular set of opportunities but also challenges to physical and mental health. Improved literacy also contributed to the proliferation of periodicals and magazines, aimed at a widening range of social classes, notably the Elementary Edu-cation Act of 1870, which standardized and enhanced educational practices for members of the working class, and improved literacy to such an extent that periodicals saw marked increases in their readerships.[10]

The periodical press also tracked and stimulated debates on questions of gender identity, ideology and practice, providing a numerous outlets for feminists and social com-mentators as well as doctors, male and female, to express their views.[11] As early as 1850, writer, theorist and advocate of women's rights, Harriet Martineau engaged with the ques-tion of healthful activities for young women, encouraging swimming and rowing, while in 1887 Dr Frances Hoggan, Medical Inspector to the North London Collegiate School for Girls, contributed to the increasingly energized debate on cycling for women, suggesting that girls could derive great benefits from cycling while also stressing that racing, competitive cycling and strenuous training was bad for women and girls.[12] Hoggan was to exemplify the cautious approach taken by a number of women doctors in advocating girls' partici-pation in education and sport, as, in her role as Medical Inspector to a leading girls' school, she traversed the complex relationships between school and home, teachers and parents, learning and exercise, and met the challenges of maintaining the well-being of pupils, many of whom—despite their relative affluence—were in a state of poor health and physique.[13]

Women formed a significant contingent of the growth in periodical readership, and many publishers introduced journals geared towards women's interests in the second half of the nineteenth century, a process coinciding with a more general feminization of the press, and the appearance of visually more enticing magazines and journals.[14] Margaret Beetham has illuminated the range and coverage of this new periodical literature for women between 1800 and 1914, demonstrating the complex and evolving engagement with their readership, and the ways that they sought to 'bring into being the women they addressed'.[15] The high-end and lavishly illustrated society journal, the *Queen*, for example, kept ladies informed on fashion and fashionable society, and also dealt with topics such as higher education for women and female employment, and advocated cycling for ladies, as well as girls clubs and gymnastics. It brought 'the concept of the lady, the techniques of illustration and the category of news into dynamic relationships with each other' and was also marked by 'an energetic, even frenetic, eclecticism'.[16] Hand in hand with the growth of periodical literature for women, the late nineteenth century was also notable for a further separation, of girls as a discrete readership with par-ticular needs and interests, an aspect of the New Journalism of the 1880s and 1890s 'with its ever more diversified target groups'.[17] And though the precise ages (and social classes) addressed by these new magazines remained elusive, as many attracted a younger and more mature readership as well as their core audience of adolescent girls, young women readers were increasingly catered for by such magazines as the *Girl's Own Paper* (*GOP*) (1880), *Young Gentlewoman* (1892), *The Girl's Realm* (1898) and *The Girl's Friend*

(1899), which included material on careers and lifestyle, health and exercise, with much of their content urging readers to engage with new ideas and activities, and instructing them on how to do so.[18]

This expanding number of periodicals, including specialist (though often short-lived) lay health journals, provided doctors who might not have had been motivated to publish full-length health guides and instructional manuals (though many did), with the opportunity to write articles and short position pieces, to contribute to advice columns and to translate their medical interests and concerns into general interest pieces, on topics such as reform clothing, hygiene and beauty, diet and abstinence, exercise and cycling, public health and the physiology of work.[19] For many, this would be a natural extension of the process of publishing in medical periodicals, as these became 'the preferred form of communication among professional men and women'.[20] A diversity of medical authors set about building a publication profile in lay periodicals—including established specialists and acknowledged leaders in their field, such as Maudsley, generalists interested in these subjects, school medical officers and women practitioners, who, like Garrett Anderson, claimed special insight into women's struggles to overcome resistance to their take-up of new and challenging roles, or, like Hoggan, exercised caution in their recommendations. Doctors were led into debates with other, often self-styled, experts on the topic of girls' health and exercise—headmistresses and teachers, gymnastics instructors, journalists and campaigners for women's rights. To a certain extent, writers on girls' health, as they debated what it consisted of and who had the right to decide this, as well as competing for copy space, vied to establish authority to instruct on and manage the process of healthful adolescence.

For many medical authors, their interest in publishing in lay outlets was inspired by a desire to raise their profile and establish their expertise in particular fields, though few were explicit in stating this objective. Many, however, declared their intentions of making an impact in the quest to improve girls' health, however they interpreted it. Physician, spiritualist and food reformer, Dr Anna Bonus Kingsford, published a series of 'Letters to Ladies' in *The Lady's Pictorial* between 1884 and 1886, which were later collected together in a volume on health and beauty for women and girls, a result, she asserted of a stream of correspondence requesting that she write such a manual. She claimed this as the first guide 'to instruct her sex on matters connected with the improvement and preservation of physical grace and good looks', taking the opportunity in addition to market a range of preparations to improve complexion and enhance the bathing experience.[21] The American physician I. P. Davis wrote a series of pieces on hygiene for girls in *Golden Hours*, a magazine for family and general consumption, in 1883, advising on amusements and exercise, nerves and the role of imagination, illuminating the growing trend for medical writers to traverse the Atlantic in their publications. While recommending a wide range of sports and healthful activities for young women, most were accompanied by warnings concerning over-exertion and access, Davis arguing that such activities should be adapted to their nature and condition.[22] Writing and publishing provided an important income stream for the redoubtable Dr Gordon Stables, prolific author of adventure stories, producer of an extensive range of health guides and health columnist for both the *GOP* and the *Boy's Own Paper*.[23] Dr Elizabeth Sloan Chesser, who, even as a medical student had earned money selling articles to local newspapers, published extensively on girls' adolescence, sexual hygiene, mothercraft and childrearing from the 1910s onwards, much of her work being aimed at a wide read-ership. As she became an established medical journalist, Chesser committed herself to pro-moting the widening access of women to professional work, careers outside the home and public life, while also urging individual responsibility for health and fitness and the impor-tance of motherhood. For Dr Mary Scharlieb, who produced numerous books and articles intended for both specialist and general readerships, women could have it all, including a professional career, but first and foremost she promoted the importance of motherhood for the national good. Youth, in her view, was a time of great instability, particularly for girls, 'whose mental powers were over-taxed' and who risked losing 'vigour and health of body'. Yet managed carefully by doctors, parents and teachers, 'the reward is great and the possibilities are great'.[24]

Increasingly periodical publications targeted particular readerships, including young women themselves. Their features also spoke directly to their readership, creating an inti-macy between author and reader though the terms 'we' or 'you' and establishing the cre-ation of good health practices as a joint concern. Dr Gordon Stables, who edited the GOP's health column for over 30 years, an ex-naval surgeon with a jaunty, straightforward, bracing, no-nonsense approach, described how 'I desire to teach my girl readers how to be healthy', as he developed a chatty (though to our eyes cloying) intimacy with his readers, including in his columns and advice books vignettes about girls who did well and those who went astray, such as Fanny Ffisher who lost her figure and found it again.[25] He concluded that the majority of the GOP's readers were 'healthy in lungs and nerves ... stout-hearted and strong-limbed'.[26] Describing how girls could further improve their strength, he provided an A to Z of dietary hints, advising morning baths and walking. 'Do not stop to stare in shop windows, but walk as if you were meant doing some-thing [sic]'.[27] 'Keep a smiling face ... fretting weakens the body'. 'The mind has much to do with the health of the body. Try to control your temper, never get angry.'[28] Stables went a long way towards defining his own girl type, his 'GOP girls', robust all-rounders, of good character but perhaps lacking somewhat in ambition: it was never quite clear what Stables actually intended his girl readers to do with their hard-won health and vitality.

Healthy girlhood was also attached to particular girl 'types' as periodical authors both created and engaged with wider trends and labels, such as the 'Girton Girl', 'a healthy young girl ... she rode, she sang, she danced, she played tennis ... she could construe one of the hardest bits of Aeschylus'.[29] The wondrous Girton Girl was, however, accompanied by other emblems of girlhood, several of whom were far from positive, bachelor girls, who sacrificed femininity to ambition and modernity, sporting types, factory girls, florid, silly and slapdash, 'The Revolting Daughter' and journalist Lynn Linton's 'Girl of the Period', who first made her appearance in the Saturday Review in 1868, and who flouted the conventions of traditional femininity, 'a creature whose sole idea of life is fun'.[30]

Among these girl types, the 'sporting girl' was framed increasingly as modern and aspirational, particularly by those with a vested interest in promoting sport for girls, adapt-ing to new urban lifestyles (for example, regularly attending a gymnasium as these sprang up in many major towns or cycling in public parks), energetic and working hard to improve her health. Catherine Horwood has noted that studying women's leisure patterns 'is a vital barometer of their ability to achieve equality', while Kathleen McCrone and Jennifer

Hargreaves have described the take-up by women and girls of physical activities and then competitive sport as challenging male exclusivity and representing feminist hopes and ambitions, as 'a new and important form of freedom', albeit one that initially was largely enjoyed by well-to-do women who could afford the associated costs and leisure time.[31]

Many doctors were eager to promote the health benefits of a well-conceived exercise culture. In 1891 Dr Alfred Schofield, Harley Street physician and prolific author on doctor–patient relationships, health practices and nervous disorders, concluded that too few girls took sufficient exercise or played enough games, which undermined their well-being, particularly against the backdrop an increasingly urbanized lifestyle: 'we confess that we consider these outdoor games and exercises necessities of almost priceless value to the population'.[32] Schofield was an intriguing figure, an active Christian, who saw the Church as having an important role in setting down the rules of life in terms of abstinence, food regimen and other health laws. He argued for the use of 'unconscious therapeutics' in his patients and the need for effective and considerate communication between doctor and patient, particularly women patients, the importance of sensitivity and listening.[33] His advice in periodicals such as *The Leisure Hour*, a journal that by virtue of its evangelical stance was a suitable outlet for Schofield, was pragmatic and generally supportive of strategies to improve girl's health and vigour, promoting a robust mental as well as physical approach (like the *GOP*, which Schofield also contributed to, *The Leisure Hour* was published by the Religious Tract Society). Hysteria's victims, he argued, were typically underworked, unhappy, suffering mental strain or exposed to an ill-balanced education; the secret of cure was 'feeling true sympathy from the conviction of the reality of the disease, but showing none'.[34] He tied the laws of health for girls not just to their general well-being but also to medical benefits and gains. He recommended exercise for health and 'firmness of limb, shapely, with well-developed muscle'. This was good for the heart, improved digestion and got rid of rheumatic and neuralgic pains. Exercise offered relief for a tired brain, and given the 'sudden increase in mental strain in the higher education of women … a safety-valve must be found in the increase in all sorts of physical pursuits'.[35]

Support for girls training and praise for sporty types would not go uncontested, far from it. In 1899, writer, physician and 'eugenic feminist', Arabella Kenealy related the story of Clara to the readers of the literary magazine *The Nineteenth Century*, which contained regular features on women's health and exercise, including the cycle craze.[36] 'A year ago Clara could not walk more than two miles without tiring; now she can play tennis or hockey, or can bicycle all day without feeling it.' Through exercise and a vigorous lifestyle, Clara had toned and honed muscles, was slimmer, stronger and more agile. However, she had also lost many of her subtle charms and qualities in the process, according to Kenealy, including sympathy and patience, and her elusive beauty. In its place a booming voice, highly toned body, a briskness, mere muscular achievement and a 'bicycle face (the face of muscular tension)'. In Kenealy's view, Clara had traded her femininity for a strident muscularity as she achieved robust health.[37] She insisted that Clara and her sister athletes were squandering 'the birthright of the babies', 'debasing her womanhood, in becoming a neuter', 'her children are nursed, fed, clothed, taught and trained by hirelings'.[38]

The Nineteenth Century then opened up the debate. Echoing the earlier controversy between Henry Maudsley and Elizabeth Garrett Anderson a decade and half earlier, the response was quick and critical, coloured by the fact that a great many girls by this time were taking to exercise rather than seeking entry to higher education in relatively small numbers. It was also inflected by eugenicist views that were shaping debates on girls' health and the proper use of their energy, and which led to broader concerns about the impact of exercise on race and nation rather than upon individual well-being. In this case, the opposition was taken up by writer and feminist, Laura Ormiston Chant, who responded in the following issue of the periodical that female athleticism would lead to the improvement and embellishment of the race rather than its decline, and that muscular vigour and moral qualities would create a nobler and happier home life for athletic girls.[39] Kenealy came back with the final say in the following issue, claiming that the stress of 'over-athletics' would lead to 'masculine women and effeminate men—neuters—spoiled copies of the human edition'. Clara herself was 'converting womanhood into mannishness by the artificial stimulation of the masculine strain in her'. The bicycle 'by reason of the exhilaration and excitement attending its use—[was] most dangerously prone to convert itself into a hobby-horse which rides its master (more still its mistress) to destruction'.[40] Physical exercise would produce, moreover, degeneration of the organs, cancer and gout; the counter to this was 'the conservation of the womanly forces. The woman whose physical completeness precludes her from spending all her energies in muscular or mental effort stores these for her children.'[41]

Kenealy's views can be contrasted with those of William Smout Playfair, Professor of Obstetric Medicine at King's College and obstetrician to King's College Hospital. Writing in a gynaecological textbook, Playfair adopted the emblem of 'Lawn Tennis Girl', lifted, as was his quotation on the benefits of tennis, from an 1895 issue of *The Speaker* magazine, to present his model of a modern, energetic girl. For Playfair, 'Lawn Tennis Girl', was

> an excellent example of the healthy, well-developed, and unsentimental girl—the girl who does not think it necessary to devote herself to the study of her own emotions, and who finds in active physical exercise an antidote to the morbid fancies which are apt to creep into the mind of the idle and self-indulgent.[42]

Clearly, for some commentators, it was the bicycle that was the problem rather than exercise more broadly, and Playfair's choice of 'Lawn Tennis Girl' to exemplify a sport that would bolster, rather than diminish, the health, well-being and femininity of girls was supported by other medical writers. One contributor to *The Practitioner* exclaimed in the same year 'it would be deplorable if girls whom lawn-tennis has made, like daughters of the gods, divinely tall should be made humpbacked by the bicycle'.[43] Dr Alfred Schofield suggested, 'There is no sight that speaks more for the future welfare of England than a group of well-made English girls returning from a tennis lawn; their every movement instinct with healthy life and vigour.'[44] Historians of sport have shown that while tennis started off as a decorous game for the affluent woman in the late nineteenth century, it gradually became a more active and energetic game, while mixed doubles, initially preserving conventional gender roles, by the interwar years incurred accusations of excessive participation and competitiveness for women players.[45]

Alfred Schofield, however, alongside his support for tennis, expressed an enthusiasm for cycling, and in a piece published in the *GOP* in 1895 explained how he had been consulted by young ladies along with their mothers to whom I felt this new exercise would prove a real boon, if used in moderation ... it develops capacity and strengthens the brain without any risk of strain ... it is no small recommendation of this new exercise that it is indubitably not only a healthy means of relieving the brain of over-pressure, but that it also exercises and strengthens this organ at the same time.[46]

Concerned to urge moderation while also counteracting the strains of an increasingly urbanized lifestyle that robbed young women of outdoor exercise, physician and public health reformer, Sir Benjamin Ward Richardson advocated cycling as a means of halting national degeneration. He reminded young women, however, that the dangers of passing 'in recreation beyond a certain bound of natural womanly duties, is to pass into a sphere with which such duties are utterly incompatible'.[47] That such views were widely held beyond the British Isles is demonstrated in Clare Simpson's article on women and cycling in late nineteenth-century New Zealand, who has illuminated the debates on respectability surrounding cycling, the importance of appropriate attire, posture and pace, and has also pointed out that issues of gender identity tended to be 'disproportionately satirized in magazines and newspapers' in relation to female cyclists.[48]

The above examples complicate our expectations about who was likely to say what about the ways in which the health of young women and challenges to it were framed by medical men. While Kenealy was a professed feminist, she was also a eugenicist, her concerns about relations between the sexes prompted chiefly 'by anxiety about the future of the British race'.[49] In her preface to fellow eugenicist, Dr Emma Walker's advice manual *Beauty Through Hygiene*, published in 1905, Kenealy warned against girls expending 'too large a share of our nervous force in athletic exercise', nerve force required for future investment in motherhood. She advised, once again, 'By habit and practice she may be able to convert herself into a mere muscular machine, but she can only do this at the expense of health and looks and qualities.'[50] Playfair, meanwhile, one of London's leading obstetric practitioners, with a lucrative private practice founded in part on the treatment of cases of neurasthenia, asserted that nerve exhaustion claimed as its victims many young women in transition from domestic to professional roles, and elsewhere expressed concern about the impact of study on young women's health. He thus put out mixed messages concerning women's ability to thrive, or, alternatively, to face physical or mental breakdown when confronted with new challenges in the schoolroom or sports field. Yet overall Playfair tended to steer a middle course, arguing for moderation, a tack taken by many medical commentators in debating the impact of education on young women. He encouraged headmistresses to pay attention to the establishment of girls' menstruation, to make proper provision for physical activity and to check that girls were not given unreasonable amounts of work or studied for excessive numbers of hours.[51]

Just as commentators on girls' health presented mixed messages, so too did the pages of host journals offer a variety of viewpoints. The *GOP* had a loose editorial regime, sometimes conservative in supporting traditional roles for women, at other times advocating new and exciting careers and sporting endeavours for its readership. In 1894 it praised modern girls for their 'strength and purpose'.[52] A year later, however, another feature, authored by none other than Dr Alfred Schofield, suggested that while the 'modern girl' had become 'stronger and more active', she was in danger of becoming physically 'overpowering', 'losing her sweeter traits', 'hard and selfish'.[53] While *The Nineteenth Century* was willing to host Kenealy's article and the exchanges that followed, three years earlier, in 1896, it had published an influential piece by Dr William Hugh Fenton that strongly promoted cycling for women, at a point where the sport was still being vigorously contested. Fenton argued that cycling might level out the difference between the sexes, allowing women to throw off some of their encumbrances, such as a dress that hampered movement and to compensate for a lack of early training: 'Women are capable of great physical improvement where the opportunity exists.' A Harley Street physician and specialist on obstetrics and gynaecology, Fenton said little on this subject in his article, focusing rather on the ways in which cycling could achieve a revolution in women's muscular tone and power, if they adopted a careful approach to build condition and endurance.[54] While space prohibits analysis of debates and recommendations concerning appropriate sporting attire for women, doctors engaged actively in such discussions, notably with regard to cycling costumes, which went beyond considerations of respectability to consider comfort, movement and hygiene. While rational dress had less of an impact in Britain, cycling clothes became looser, lighter, warmer and more practical, with shorter skirts worn over knickerbockers. 'Lady Doctor', Miss Crosfield, recommended abandoning corsets and wearing wide shoes for comfort, Gordon Stables urged 'the fair rider' to follow the example of men who exercise, and, on returning home, to bathe and change their clothing, and both urged the adoption of woollen underwear.[55]

Gordon Stables' publications reflect the ways in which individual author's opinions could also change over time, and in his case apparently dovetail with eugenicist ideas and language in the build-up of anxieties about race, nation and Empire at the turn of the century. Stables appeared to subscribe to a straightforward vision of the 'fixed fund of energy' thesis during the 1880s and 1890s, recognizing the scope for incremental improvement in physique and well-being in all young women: 'All kinds of exercise do good; walking for the weakly, cycling and rowing for the stronger, dumb-bells and Indian clubs before breakfast or in the afternoon for all.'[56] Though he was cautious concerning the benefits of cycling for girls, especially those under the age of 15, and encouraged weaker girls to use a tricycle, he lauded the cycle's overall health benefits.[57] But by 1901, likely spurred on by the stepping up of Empire rhetoric in the midst of the South African War, Stables' views shifted, and his readers warned not to 'have too much of that emancipation business'. 'Who wants a woman with biceps, anyhow?'[58] His earlier publications had encouraged girls not to stand on the sidelines but to join in the sporting endeavours of their brothers. Now he denounced girls' pursuit of 'man-games and tomboy exercises' that would result in their loss of womanly elegance. Golf would lead to the 'ungainly and hoydenish golf stride', while hockey 'was the most hoydenish and ungraceful of all man-games and soon gains for her a figure with not more grace in it than of an oyster-wife'.[59] In a reversal of his earlier modest support of cycling for girls, and nudging close to Kenealy's assessment of the sport, he described how biking

> Rolls the spine, interferes with the proper function of the hip-bones and gives the bicycle face, with its 'blintering' eyes, look of deep concern, square jaws and flabby mock-turtle cheeks. It is nice to be able to move quickly about in this age of hurry, but biking is after all but a man-game.[60]

Just as youth itself, particularly girls' youth, was seen as fluid, complex and a time of opportunities and challenges, so too was girls' healthy passage through it complex and much debated.[61] For many medical authors, like Stables, attitudes hardened by the early twentieth century, as medical ideas and literature became imbued with notions of national efficiency, which were replicated in wider interest periodicals. Such periodicals presented diverse views on the limits of education and physical exertion, demonstrating the capacity of their authors and editors to contribute to both the reproduction and construction of ideas on gender and health. The impact of all this writing is difficult to measure, not least given the diversity of the viewpoints expressed by doctors—which were not neatly divided by gender or even consistent for individual authors—and the challenges of assessing what lay readers, including women and girls, actually made of medicine's efforts to inform and instruct on matters pertaining to their health. The apparent marketability of such advice literature and the enduring popularity of the health column and articles on exercise and health intended for women and girl readers indicates, however, that they were exposed extensively to such materials in a range of general interest and specialist periodicals. What all this activity also illuminated is the eagerness of doctors to disseminate their views broadly, via an ever-expanding and editorially flexible periodical literature, and to engage actively with the issues of the day, relating health and health practices to major cultural and social changes.

Disclosure Statement

No potential conflict of interest was reported by the author.

Notes

1. Explored in Marland, *Health and Girlhood*; this article focuses on the ways in which doctors and other self-styled authorities on girls' health utilized periodical literature to convey their opinions.
2. Anon., "Women's Beauty." The article summarized eminent psychiatrist Sir James Crichton-Browne's take on the challenges of female education for women.
3. Flint, *The Woman Reader*, 57.
4. Scull, MacKenzie, and Hervey, "Degeneration and Despair"; Turner, "Henry Maudsley"; Brock, *British Women Surgeons*; Manton, *Elizabeth Garrett Anderson*; and Elston, "Anderson, Elizabeth Garrett."
5. Maudsley, "Sex in Mind."
6. Vertinsky, *The Eternally Wounded Woman*, 46.
7. Anderson, "Sex in Mind."
8. Flint, *The Woman Reader*, 57. For the debate and its follow-up, see Burstyn, "Education and Sex"; Newman, *Men's Ideas/Women's Realities*; and Marland, *Health and Girlhood*, ch. 4.
9. Vann and VanArsdel, *Victorian Periodicals*, 3, 7–8.
10. Van Vuuren, *Literary Research*, 145.
11. Fraser, Green, and Johnston, *Gender and the Victorian Periodical*.
12. Martineau, "How to Learn to Swim"; Hoggan, "Cycling for Ladies."

13. Marland, *Health and Girlhood*, 122–31, and for the contributions of medical practitioners to the debate on cycling 103–18.

14. See also Parratt, "Athletic 'Womanhood'," 43.

15. Beetham, *A Magazine of Her Own?*, preface, ix.

16. Ibid., 89, 91.

17. Ibid., 138. See also Drotner, *English Children*; Tinkler, *Constructing Girlhood*; and Mitchell, *The New Girl*.

18. For the *Girl's Own Paper* (*GOP*), see Skelding, "Every Girls' Best Friend?"; Drotner, *English Children*, ch. 10; Marland, *Health and Girlhood*, 75–82; and Beetham, *A Magazine of Her Own?*, ch. 9.

19. Peterson, "Medicine."

20. Vann and VanArsdel, *Victorian Periodicals*, 5.

21. Kingsford, *Health, Beauty and the Toilet*. See also Richardson, "Transforming the Body Politic."

22. Davis, "Hygiene for Girls," 655–60. See also Verbrugge, *Able-Bodied Womanhood*, 121–2.

23. See Marland, *Health and Girlhood*, 51–2, 75–82 for Stables' publishing exploits and the *GOP*.

24. Scharlieb, "Adolescent Girlhood," 179; Scharlieb, "Adolescent Girls," 1015. See Jones, "Women and Eugenics in Britain."

25. Stables, *The Girl's Own Book*, preface, 174–82.

26. 'Medicus', "The Weather and Health," 23–4.

27. 'Medicus', "Can Girls Increase their Strength?" 534.

28. 'Medicus', "Health, Strength and Beauty," 758; 'Medicus', "Health All the Year Round," 166.

29. Mitchell, *The New Girl*, 65, for citation of Nesbit, E. 'The Girton Girl', *Atalanta* 8 (1895), 755–759, on 755.

30. Anon. [Linton, E. Lynn], "The Girl of the Period," *Saturday Review* 25 (March 14, 1868), 339–340. Reprinted in Linton, *The Girl of the Period*, 6, 2. See also Fraser, Green, and Johnston, *Gender and the Victorian Periodical*, 32–4 for the complex gender formations taking place in *Girl of the Period Miscellany*.

31. Horwood, "Girls Who Arouse Dangerous Passions," 654; McCrone, *Sport and the Physical Emancipation*; Hargreaves, *Sporting Females*, 42. See also Macrae, *Exercise in the Female Life Cycle*, ch. 3 for the experiences of young girls after 1930.

32. Schofield, "The Modern Development," 818.

33. Imber, *Trusting Doctors*, 85–7.

34. Schofield, "Nervousness and Hysteria," 415.

35. Schofield, "Modern Hygiene in Practice," 672, 673.

36. See Marland, *Health and Girlhood*, ch. 3.

37. Kenealy, "Woman as Athlete," 635, 641.

38. Ibid., 643, 645.

39. Chant, "Woman as an Athlete."

40. Kenealy, "Woman as an Athlete: A Rejoinder," 916, 920.

41. Ibid., 924, 926, 928.

42. Playfair, "The Nervous System," 221. Playfair was citing a leading article, 'The New Woman – Old Style', *The Speaker* (January 12, 1895), 39–41, on 40.

43. Anon., "The Month," 111.

44. Schofield, "The Modern Development," 818.

45. Hargreaves, *Sporting Females*, 54–5, Lake, "Gender and Etiquette in British Lawn Tennis," 703–4.
46. Schofield, "The Cycling Craze," 185.
47. Richardson, "On Recreation for Girls," 546.
48. Simpson, "Respectable Identities," 69, 68.
49. Richardson, "Arabella Madonna Kenealy."
50. Walker, *Beauty Through Hygiene*, preface, 10, 11.
51. Playfair, "Remarks on the Education."
52. F.H. [Hird], "Women's Work," 51.
53. Schofield, "On the Perfecting," 662.
54. Fenton, "A Medical View of Cycling," 797.
55. Anon., "A Lady Doctor on Cycling"; Stables, *Girls' Own Book*, 62. For dress reform and sport, see McCrone, *Sport and the Physical Emancipation*, ch. 8.
56. 'Medicus', "A Plain Talk," 597.
57. Stables, *Health upon Wheels*, 43.
58. Stables ('Medicus'), "Health," 716.
59. Stables ('Medicus'), "Man-Games," 503.
60. Ibid., 503.
61. See also Marland, "Unstable Adolescence."

Bibliography

Anderson, Elizabeth Garrett. "Sex in Mind and Education: A Reply." *The Fortnightly Review* 15 (May 1874): 582–594.

Anon. "The Month." *The Practitioner* 55 (August 1895): 111.

Anon. "Women's Beauty." *Good Health* VIII, no. 188 (May 9, 1896): 170–171.

Anon. "A Lady Doctor on Cycling." *Hub* (September 26, 1896): 287(Modern Records Centre, University of Warwick, National Cycle Archive: MSS 328/C/5/HUB).

Beetham, Margaret. *A Magazine of Her Own? Domesticity and Desire in the Woman's Magazine, 1800–1914*. London: Routledge, 1996.

Brock, Claire. *British Women Surgeons and Their Patients, 1860–1918*. Cambridge: Cambridge University Press, 2017.

Burstyn, Joan. "Education and Sex: The Medical Case Against Higher Education in England, 1870–1900." *Proceedings of the American Philosophical Society* 117 (1973): 79–89.

Chant, L. Ormiston. "Woman as an Athlete: A Reply to Dr Arabella Kenealy." *The Nineteenth Century* (May 1899): 915–919.

Davis, I. P. "Hygiene for Girls. Amusements." *Golden Hours: A Monthly Magazine for Family and General Reading* (November 1883): 665–660.

Drotner, Kirsten. *English Children and Their Magazines, 1751–1945*. New Haven, CT: Yale University Press, 1988.

Elston, M. A. "Anderson, Elizabeth Garrett (1836–1917)." In *Dictionary of National Biography*. Accessed September 1, 2016. http://0-www.oxforddnb.com.pugwash.lib.warwick.ac.uk/view/article/30406.

Fenton, W. H. "A Medical View of Cycling for Ladies." *The Nineteenth Century* (January–June 1896): 796–801.

Flint, Kate. *The Woman Reader 1837–1914*. Oxford: Clarendon, 1993.

Fraser, Hilary, Stephanie Green, and Judith Johnston. *Gender and the Victorian Periodical*. Cambridge: Cambridge University Press, 2003.

Hargreaves, Jennifer. *Sporting Females: Critical Issues in the History and Sociology of Women's Sports*. London: Routledge, 1994.

H., F. [Hird, Frank]. "Women's Work: Its Value and Possibilities." *Girl's Own Paper* XVI, no. 774 (October 27, 1894): 51.

Hoggan, Francis Elizabeth. "Cycling for Ladies" (Correspondence). *Cyclists' Touring Club Gazette* (December 1887): 454. (Modern Records Centre, University of Warwick, National Cycle Archive: MSS.328/C/4/CYT).

Horwood, Catherine. "'Girls Who Arouse Dangerous Passions': Women and Bathing, 1900–1939." *Women's History Review* 9 (2000): 653–673.

Imber, Jonathan B. *Trusting Doctors: The Decline of Moral Authority in American Medicine*. Princeton, NJ: Princeton University Press, 2008.

Jones, Greta. "Women and Eugenics in Britain: The Case of Mary Scharlieb, Elizabeth Sloan Chesser, and Stella Browne." *Annals of Science* 52 (1995): 481–502.

Kenealy, Arabella. April 1899. "Woman as Athlete." *The Nineteenth Century* 635–645.

Kenealy, Arabella. "Woman as an Athlete: A Rejoinder." *The Nineteenth Century* (June 1899): 915–929.

Kingsford, Anna Bonus. *Health, Beauty and the Toilet: Letters to Ladies from a Lady Doctor*. London: Frederick Warne, 1886.

Lake, Robert J. "Gender and Etiquette in British Lawn Tennis 1870–1939: A Case Study of 'Mixed Doubles'." *The International Journal of the History of Sport* 29 (2012): 691–710.

Linton, E. Lynn. *The Girl of the Period and Other Social Essays*. Vol. 1. London: Richard Bentley, 1883.

Macrae, Eilidh. *Exercise in the Female Life-Cycle in Britain 1930–1970*. Houndmills: Palgrave Macmillan, 2016.

Manton, Jo. *Elizabeth Garrett Anderson*. London: Methuen, 1965.

Marland, Hilary. *Health and Girlhood in Britain, 1874–1920*. Houndmills: Palgrave Macmillan, 2013.

Marland, Hilary. "Unstable Adolescence/Unstable Literature? Managing British Girls' Health Around 1900." In *Picturing Women's Health*, edited by Francesca Scott, Kate Scarth, and Ji Won Chung, 159–172. London: Pickering and Chatto, 2014.

Martineau, Harriet. "How to Learn to Swim." *Once a Week* 1, no. 16 (1859): 327–328.

Maudsley, Henry. "Sex in Mind and in Education." *The Fortnightly Review* 15 (April 1874): 466–483.

McCrone, Kathleen E. *Sport and the Physical Emancipation of English Women 1870–1914*. London: Routledge, 1988.

'Medicus'. "Health All the Year Round." *Girl's Own Paper* VI, no. 259 (December 13, 1884): 166–167.

'Medicus'. "The Weather and Health." *Girl's Own Paper* VIII, no. 354 (October 9, 1886): 23–24.

'Medicus'. "Health, Strength and Beauty." *Girl's Own Paper* XI, no. 557 (August 30, 1890): 758–759.

'Medicus'. "Can Girls Increase Their Strength?" *Girl's Own Paper* XV, no. 752 (May 26, 1894): 534.

'Medicus'. "A Plain Talk with Sensible Girls." *Girl's Own Paper* XVII, no. 860 (June 20, 1896): 597.

Mitchell, Sally. *The New Girl: Girls' Culture in England 1880–1915*. New York: Columbia University Press, 1995.

Newman, Louise Michelle. *Men's Ideas/Women's Realities: Popular Science, 1870–1915.* New York: Permagon, 1985.

Parratt, Catriona M. "Athletic 'Womanhood': Exploring Sources for Female Sport in Victorian and Edwardian England." *Journal of Sport History* 16 (1989): 40–52.

Peterson, M. Jeanne. "Medicine." In *Victorian Periodicals and Victorian Society*, edited by J. Don Vann and Rosemary T. VanArsdel, 22–44. Aldershot: Scolar, 1994.

Playfair, W. S. "Remarks on the Education and Training of Girls of the Easy Classes at and about the Period of Puberty." *British Medical Journal* 2 (December 7, 1895): 1408–1410.

Playfair, W. S. "The Nervous System in Relation to Gynaecology." In *A System of Gynaecology by Many Writers*, edited by T. C. Allbutt and W. S. Playfair, 220–232. London: Macmillan, 1896.

Richardson, Angelique. "Arabella Madonna Kenealy (1859–1938)." In Dictionary of National Biography. Accessed September 1, 2016. http://0-www.oxforddnb.com.pugwash.lib.warwick.ac.uk/view/article/50057

Richardson, Sir Benjamin Ward. "On Recreation for Girls." *Girl's Own Paper* XV, no. 753 (June 2, 1894): 545–547.

Richardson, Sarah. "Transforming the Body Politic: Food Reform and Feminism in Nineteenth-Century Britain." In *Picturing Women's Health*, edited by Francesca Scott, Kate Scarth, and Ji Won Chung, 45–57. London: Pickering and Chatto, 2014.

Scharlieb, Mary. "Adolescent Girlhood under Modern Conditions, with a Special Reference to Motherhood." *The Eugenics Review* 1 (1909): 174–183.

Scharlieb, Mary A. D. "Adolescent Girls from the Viewpoint of the Physician." *The Child* 1, no. 12 (September 1911): 1013–1031.

Schofield, Alfred. "Modern Hygiene in Practice." *The Leisure Hour* (August 1894): 670–675.

Schofield, A. T. December 21, 1895. "The Cycling Craze." *Girl's Own Paper* XVII (834): 185–186.

Schofield, A. T. June 1, 1895. "On the Perfecting of the Modern Girl." *Girl's Own Paper* XVI (805): 662.

Schofield, A. T. "Nervousness and Hysteria." *The Leisure Hour* (June 1889): 412–415.

Schofield, Alfred T. "The Modern Development of Athletics." *The Leisure Hour* (October 1891): 817–820.

Scull, Andrew, Charlotte MacKenzie, and Nicholas Hervey. "Degeneration and Despair: Henry Maudsley, (1835–1918)." In *Masters of Bedlam: The Transformation of the Mad-Doctoring Trade*, edited by Andrew Scull, Charlotte MacKenzie, and Nicholas Hervey, 226–267. Princeton, NJ: Princeton University Press, 1996.

Skelding, Hilary. "Every Girls' Best Friend? The *Girl's Own Paper* and Its Readers." In *Feminist Readings of Victorian Popular Texts: Divergent Femininities*, edited by Emma Liggins and Daniel Duffy, 35–52. Aldershot: Ashgate, 2001.

Stables, Gordon. *Health upon Wheels; or, Cycling a Means of Maintaining the Health.* London: Iliffe, 1887.

Stables, Gordon. *The Girl's Own Book of Health and Beauty.* London: Jarrold, 1891.

Stables, Gordon ('Medicus'). "Health." *Girl's Own Paper* XXII, no. 1128 (August 10, 1901): 716–717.

Stables, Gordon ('Medicus'). "Man-Games That Murder Beauty." *Girl's Own Paper* XXVII, no. 1376 (May 12, 1906): 502–503.

Tinkler, Penny. *Constructing Girlhood: Popular Magazines for Girls Growing up in England 1920–1950.* London: Taylor & Francis, 1995.

Turner, T. H. "Henry Maudsley (1835–1918)." In *Dictionary of National Biography*. Accessed September 1, 2016. http://0-www.oxforddnb.com.pugwash.lib.warwick.ac.uk/view/article/37747.

Turner, Mark. "Hybrid Journalism: Women and the Progressive Fortnightly." In *Journalism, Literature and Modernity: From Hazlitt to Modernism*, edited by Kate Campbell, 72–90. Edinburgh: Edinburgh University Press, 2000.

Vann, J. Don, and Rosemary T. VanArsdel, eds. *Victorian Periodicals and Victorian Society*. Aldershot: Scolar, 1994.

Van Vuuren, Melissa S. *Literary Research and the Victorian and Edwardian Ages, 1830–1910: Strategies and Sources*. Lanham, MD: Scarecrow, 2011.

Verbrugge, Martha H. *Able-Bodied Womanhood: Personal Health and Social Change in Nineteenth-Century Boston*. New York: Oxford University Press, 1997.

Vertinsky, Patricia A. 1994. *The Eternally Wounded Woman: Women, Doctors, and Exercise in the Late Nineteenth Century*. Urbana, IL: University of Illinois Press. 1st published Manchester University Press, 1989.

Walker, Emma E. *Beauty Through Hygiene: Commonsense Ways to Health for Girls*. London: Hutchinson, 1905.

USING DIGITISED MEDICAL JOURNALS IN A CROSS EUROPEAN PROJECT ON ADDICTION HISTORY

Alex Mold and **Virginia Berridge**

This article draws on research conducted as part of a European project on the changing terminology used to conceptualise habitual drug, alcohol or tobacco use. We wanted to find out what language was utilised in Italy, Poland, Austria and the UK and how those concepts had changed since the mid-nineteenth century. We intended to make use of digitised journals for key word searches to enable comparisons to be made across countries and across time. Nothing, however, was straightforward. Few countries had digitised medical journals, so researchers had to use traditional search methods. Even in the UK, where journals were available digitally, there were problems with access and the searches that could be made. Digitisation did not provide a quicker way of researching cross nationally. Nonetheless our work did arrive at some valuable new conclusions. Our experiences also raise wider questions about using digitised journals for historical research.

Introduction

In recent years much ink (both real and electronic) has been spilled on the opportunities and drawbacks presented by the digitisation of historical sources. Previously hard to obtain resources have been made more accessible and new tools, such as text mining, allow researchers to conduct searches in minutes rather than over many months or years. Published sources like newspapers and periodicals are some of the most commonly digitised sources, and the nineteenth century is a period that is particularly well served by digitisation projects.[1] Whilst there are a plethora of possibilities offered by the 'digital turn', the revolution is far from complete, and there are many issues still to be resolved.[2] In this article we explore some of the advantages and disadvantages of attempting to make use of digitised medical journals, especially when working cross-nationally. Drawing on research conducted as part of a European project on the changing terminology used to conceptualise habitual drug, alcohol or tobacco use, we highlight some of the problems presented by digitised sources but also point to ways in which this kind of research generated new and unexpected insights. Our findings were novel within the history of substance use, but also raise questions about digitisation projects and the ways in which historians make use of these.

This article is divided into three sections. We begin by detailing the wider project of which this research was part, and setting it the context of the existing literature on the history of substance use. Our findings come from work conducted as part of a European Union Framework Programme 7 funded project on addiction across Europe. The Addiction Lifestyles in Contemporary Europe: Reframing Addictions Project (ALICE RAP) brought together a range of researchers from different disciplines and European countries to address the problems associated with substance use and addictive behaviours. One of the ALICE RAP workpackages, 'Addiction Through the Ages', focused specifically on the history of addiction across Europe, a largely under-explored topic within the history of substance use. In the second section of the article, we discuss in more detail our methodology for researching the history of addiction in Europe during the nineteenth century, and the ways in which we attempted to make use of digitised medical journals. We encountered a number of problems, some of which were due to the sources themselves, but others were related to our cross-national focus. We found that digitisation programmes were not always so advanced in the other European countries within our project, forcing us to resort to more traditional search methods. Moreover, the changing nature of both our topic of research (the terminology surrounding drug, alcohol and tobacco use) and the fluctuating borders of the European countries we focused on, presented us with several moving targets. In the third section of the article we discuss some of the findings from our research. Our exploration of the language of addiction over the period 1860–1930 in different European countries (Austria, Italy, Poland and the UK) generated novel data, and goes some way to correcting an Anglo-American bias in the history of substance use. The research also threw up several interesting questions about doing digital research when working across different countries and time periods. We reflect on these issues in the conclusion, arguing that historians, archivists, librarians and funders need to work together to make sources available and usable for future generations of researchers.

The ALICE RAP Project: Addiction Through the Ages Across Europe

The ALICE RAP project was a five-year research collaboration running from 2011–2016 with a vision 'to promote well being through a synthesis of knowledge to redesign European policy and practice to better address the challenges posed by substance use and addictive behaviours'.[3] The project was large, with seven broad areas and twenty-one workpackages. Over 200 researchers were involved from twenty-five countries and twenty-nine disciplines. The history workpackage was led by Professor Virginia Berridge. Findings from this research and other parallel projects have been published in several articles and collated in an edited volume on concepts of addictive substances and behaviours over time and space.[4] The history workpackage was set up to involve a collection of pre-existing partners from pre-selected European countries. Partners in this component of the workpackage came from the UK; Austria; Italy; and Poland. Although these case-studies countries were pre-selected (as part of the way the wider ALICE RAP project was designed) they represented a good mix of geography, comprising of countries from Western, Central, Southern and Eastern Europe, with different cultural attitudes towards, and histories of, substance use.

The core purpose of the history workpackage was to chart the changing terminology of addiction over the course of the period between 1860 and 1980. A broad framework for the project was established before we began the research, and we developed a more specific programme of action once the research was underway. We began by breaking this period into three phases: the 1860s–1930s, the 1950s–1960s, and finally the 1970s–1980s. We chose these periods as the existing historiography suggested that these were eras when changes in the concepts used to describe substance use may have occurred. The late nineteenth and early twentieth centuries, (as we discuss in greater detail below) were a time when the concept of 'addiction' in relation to drugs and alcohol was established and elaborated. We thought that the period from the 1950s-1960s would also be of interest, as this was when international organisations, such as the World Health Organisation, began to play a role in describing and responding to addiction. Our final phase, from the 1970s to the 1980s, was a period when drug and alcohol problems grew in size and scale, and we wanted to see what impact this had on the terminology used to describe them.

But, as we shall see, we encountered a number of practical and conceptual difficulties in our attempt to use digitised sources. Although this may be of no surprise to experienced digital researchers, it is an important point to reiterate, as it raises wider questions about how non-experts in using digitised sources approach these and how these are used in conjunction with non-digitised material, especially when working cross-nationally.

Carrying out historical work on addiction across and within European countries was particularly important, as though there is a vibrant literature on drugs, alcohol and tobacco use, much of this is focused on the USA and the UK. With some notable exceptions, research has tended to centre on substance use in an Anglo-American context.[5] A particular area of interest surrounds the emergence and development of the concept of 'addiction'. For some observers, such as the historian Jessica Warner, the modern disease-based concept of alcohol addiction first appeared in the seventeenth century. She contended that Stuart clergymen often described habitual drunkenness in terms of addiction. Other historians, like Roy Porter, place the origins of the concept of addiction in the eighteenth century.[6] A disease-based concept of addiction can be observed in the work of Benjamin Rush in America and Thomas Trotter in England towards the end of the eighteenth century.[7] During the nineteenth century, the notion of addiction underwent significant change, as the growing forces of evangelism and urbanisation gave the concept of addiction new weight. The appearance of the temperance movement, and the need for doctors to explain the overwhelming desire for drink, helped to consolidate an understanding of addiction that located the problem in the drink rather than the drinker. The word 'alcoholism', first developed by Magnus Huss in Sweden, began to come in to use as a distinct term to describe disease-based understandings of compulsive alcohol use.

In the nineteenth century, disease-based understandings of addiction expanded to include other substances as well as alcohol. New and more potent drugs, more effective methods of administration and medical professional involvement, drove this development. Addiction came to be seen as a 'disease of the will', an understanding that combined both medical and moral elements.[8] Such a view could be found in the arguments of temperance reformers and anti-opium campaigners as well in the medical literature. This medico-moral alliance was part of a wider trend that saw other issues, such as madness and sexuality, in a similar light. All of this is not to say, however, that tension did not exist between medical and moral approaches. As Mariana Valverde has demonstrated, medico-moral discord meant that there was no universally agreed definition of addiction, and no universally accepted treatment for the condition either.[9]

Indeed, it is striking that during the nineteenth and twentieth centuries there were a range of terms in use to denote addiction to alcohol and other psychoactive substances.

The term 'inebriety' features centrally within the Anglo-American literature of the time, a word that covered addiction to both drink and drugs. The development of the concept of inebriety was connected to the work of professional societies, such as the British Society for the Study and Cure of Inebriety, which was established in 1884.[10] The notion of inebriety offered an alternative to the criminalisation of the drinker, allowing for the treatment, rather than the incarceration, of inebriates. Yet other words, like 'alcoholism', were also employed to describe habitual problems associated with substance use. What led to the emergence and development of these terms, and how did their usage and meanings change over the course of the nineteenth century and early twentieth century? Moreover, were these terms confined to the UK and the US, or were they used in Continental Europe too? How did imported concepts interact with the pre-existing domestic language to describe substance use? What were the origins of these terms, and how were they similar or different to the words used in the other countries within the study?

Methodological Challenges and Approaches in Researching the Cross-national History of Addiction Concepts

In order to answer such questions we agreed, together with our European partners, to design a common methodology to chart the changing terminology of addiction. For our first period (1860s–1930s), we agreed that we would focus on the medical approach to substance use, and make use of digitised medical journals where possible.[11] For our second (1950s-1960s) and third (1970s-1980s) periods we took a different tack. We decided to move away from the focus on medical texts to look at how addiction concepts were utilised within policy documents produced in these decades.[12] All of the researchers in the different countries (Austria, Italy, Poland and the UK) agreed to adopt this common methodology, so that as far as possible our results would be comparable. We decided that this could be achieved by examining one general medical journal, one specialist addiction journal, and one medical textbook for each country. We knew that the medical textbooks were unlikely to be digitised, but we assumed naïvely that the digitisation of medical journals in the UK would make this part of the research relatively straightforward and quick to generate results both for the British study, and for our European partners. The full results of our research based on this approach are summarised elsewhere, but here we concentrate on the work we did with the medical journals. Based on the existing historiography, we collated a list of terms used to describe drug and alcohol use in English (Table 1), which we then intended to search for in the digitised medical journals. We wanted to count how frequently the different terms were used in the medical journals and plot any changes and continuities over time. We also wanted to see if these terms were translated into the different languages used in or study countries, or if these countries had their own terminology to describe drug and alcohol problems.

Operationalising this approach, however, proved more difficult than we thought. There were a number of issues around how to translate the search terms from English into the different European languages used in our study countries. For some terms, there was an obvious English equivalent: 'Alcoholism', for instance, could be translated into 'Alkoholizm' in Polish; 'Alkoholismus' in German and 'Alcolismo' in Italian. But even here there were differences, (as we explore in more detail below) in Austria 'Alkoholismus'

TABLE 1.
English key word search terms

English Key Word Search Terms
Habit
Dipsomania
Alcoholism
Chronic Poisoning
Morphinomania
Narcomania
Inebriety
Morphinism
Addiction

did not enjoy the conceptual hegemony experienced elsewhere in Europe, as there was another set of terms around drink and the drinker that were also in use. Moreover, other words proved to be untranslatable, or local differences in meaning implied that terms could not be considered synonymous. 'Addiction' for example, could be translated as 'Nałóg' in Polish, but the term could be used as both a noun and an adjective (Table 2).

There were practical problems too. We thought that each country would have its own general medical journal, and a more specialist publication devoted to drug and alcohol use (as in the UK). This was not the case in any of our Continental European focus countries. In Italy, there was no general medical journal in this period, so the researchers had to focus on more specialist publications, particularly in forensic science.[13] In Poland, researchers could not find a specialist journal that dealt with substance use, but there were two general medical journals, one that was published weekly and another monthly. Records of the monthly journal, however, were incomplete, especially during the period of the Polish-Soviet War (1918–21).[14] In Austria, the situation was further complicated by the fact that the language used did not coincide with the national border. German was the language of the republic as well as the Empire, and spoken in the neighbouring countries where most of the medical journals were published (Table 3).[15]

More fundamentally, few of the European journals had been digitised. When we began the project none of them had, but during the course of our research some of the Polish journals became available digitally, although these were incomplete with large gaps. So, our European colleagues largely had to rely on hand sorting and counting to locate addiction terminology. Not only was this much more time consuming (a significant issue when a fixed amount of time and resources could be devoted to the research) but it also required the research teams in the different countries to take slightly different approaches. The Austrian researcher decided that a differentiation needed to be made between the use of addiction terms in 'short' and 'main' articles; the Italian team used the journal index and contents pages to identify relevant articles, and then counted the number of addiction terms used within these articles; the Polish team counted the number of 'units' (articles, letters, short reports and notes) that referred to substance use and the different terminology used.[16] Specificities in each of the countries within the study thus resulted in a dilution of the common research method. This made direct comparison between the different countries more difficult, but general trends did emerge.

TABLE 2.
Terms used to describe drug & alcohol use in European study countries

Country	Terms used	English translation
Austria	Alkoholismus	Alcoholism
	Trunkenheit	Intoxication
	Trunksuch	Ailing due to drinking
	Gewohnheitsstrinker	Habitual drinker
Italy	Alcolismo	Alcoholism
	Avvelenamento da alcol	Alcohol poisoning
	Delirium tremens	Delirium Tremens
	Dipsomania	Dipsomania
	Intossicazione alcolica	Alcohol intoxication
	Psicosi alcoliche	Alcoholic psychosis
	Ubriachezza	Drunkenness
	Ubriachezza abituale	Habitual drunkenness
	Ubriachezza patologica	Pathological drunkenness
	Avvelenamento da morfina	Morphine poisoning
	Morfinismo	Morphinism
	Morfinodipsia	Morphine dipsomania
	Morfinomania	Morphinomania
	Avvelenamento da cocaina	Cocaine poisoning
	Cocainismo	Cocainism
	Intossicazione da cocaina	Cocaine intoxication
	Avvelenamento da eroina	Heroin poisoning
	Avvelenamento da oppio	Opium poisoning
	Intossicazione da nicotina	Nicotine intoxication
	Intossicazione da tabacco	Tobacco intoxication
	Nicotinismo	Nicotinism
Poland	Alkoholizm	Alcoholism
	Dipsomania, dypsomania	Dipsomania
	Kokainizm	Cocainism
	Morfinizm	Morphinism
	Nałóg	Addiction
	Nałogowy pijak	Addicted drunkard
	Narkomania	Drug addiction
	Nawyk	Habit
	Nikotynizm	Nicotinism
	Opilstwo	Inebriety
	Pijaństwo	Drunkenness
	Tytomania	Tobacco addiction
	Zatrucie, przewlekłe i ostre	Poisoning, chronic and acute

Even in the UK, where digital versions of our chosen sources—the *British Medical Journal (BMJ)*, *The Lancet* and the *British Journal of Inebriety*—were obtainable, there were problems. The journals were all digitised, with searchable online archives and articles available as pdf. files. But, to our surprise, this did not necessarily mean ease of access and analysis. Each journal was available under a different licensing agreement and this constrained our ability to conduct keyword searches. The *British Journal of Inebriety* required a user subscription, whilst full-text electronic access to the *Lancet* was only available onsite at two libraries. The *BMJ* and *Lancet* covered the whole of our time period from 1860 to 1930, but only post-1904 search results could be obtained for the *British Journal of Inebriety*. The journal's predecessor, *Proceedings*, was available as scanned (jpeg.) images, but this

TABLE 3.
Journals used by country

Country	Journals Used
Austria	*Wiener Medizinische Wochenschrift* (general medical journal); *Jahrbücher für Psychatrie/ Jahrbücher für Psychiatrie und Neurologie* (specialist psychiatritc journal)
Italy	*Archives of Criminal Anthropology, Psychiatry, Forensic Science and related Science; Experimental Journal of Psychiatry and Forensic Science of the Mental Alienation; Journal of Forensic Science; Journal of Forensic Science; Journal of Forensic Science and Medical Jurisprudence* (all forensic science journals)
Poland	*Gazeta lekarska (Physician's Gazette); Nowiny lekarskie (Medical News)* (all general medical journals)
UK	*British Medical Journal; The Lancet* (general medical journals) *British Journal of Inebriety* (specialist journal)

prevented comparable electronic searches without the aid of text recognition software and analysis could only be done on a page by page basis, a very laborious activity.

Once we had access, using the digitised sources to conduct the keyword searches also proved to be problematic. The way in which some of the journals had been digitised and made available impeded our research. For example, the default search option with some sources included all a publisher's titles rather than allowing a search within a specific time frame and journal. Creating a search that focused on just one journal was complicated and time consuming as the other journals needed to be manually filtered out. Furthermore, it was not always possible to sort search results in order. This posed a particular challenge for terms that produced a large amount of results. Key-word searches within electronic articles were also inconsistent, and sometimes failed to capture terms within the text, especially when the file resolution was poor. Our chosen search terms also caused some difficulties. Words like 'habit' could be applied in many contexts, thus generating false positives in the results. Furthermore, the inclusion of 'inebriety' in a journal name, and the widely documented creation of the 'Society of the Study of Inebriety' (1884) both presented further difficulties, over emphasising the use of the term. Finally, certain words yielded insufficient data, which impeded attempts to chart their changing usage over time, or to make meaningful comparisons with how and when they were used in the other literature. Digitisation, then, was not a route to the quick and easy generation of results.

Addiction Terminology in Europe, 1860s–1930s

Despite these many difficulties, we were able to acquire some useful data and use this to gain a new insight into addiction and its terminology in Europe during the period 1860–1930. Overall, the research showed considerable divergences between countries in this period but also some significant points of convergence. We will summarise the results of our work in this period by country and then discuss them overall.[17] In the UK, the digital searches showed very clearly the rise and predominance of the concept of inebriety in the medical arena from the 1870s. There were, for instance, 4 uses of 'inebriety' in the *BMJ* in 1878, rising to 32 by 1890. Further periods of extensive debate occurred in the 1900s, at a time of discussion of the extension of inebriates legislation and concerns about national degeneration. Usage of 'inebriety' peaked in 1902 in the *Lancet* and 1914 in the *BMJ*, with just less than 90 usages of the term in each journal in each year. But the term fell out of favour at the time of the First World War and was rarely used thereafter. Two terms began to replace the unified inebriety concept. One was 'alcoholism' and the other was 'addiction'. The former term began to rise in prominence from the late nineteenth century but it did not achieve acceptability in the way in which 'drug addiction' did and declined after the First World War, perhaps in line with reduced interest in alcohol as a social issue in the inter-war years. The term 'alcoholism' was used 11 times in 1884 in the *BMJ*, rising to a peak of 88 times in 1914, but fell rapidly after this so that the term only occurred 9 times by 1919. 'Addiction', however, began its rise after 1918. The term was virtually unused before this date, but incidences of usage increased rapidly. By 1922 it occurred seven times in the *BMJ* and 16 times by 1927.

These patterns were representative of a significant divergence from ways of describing habitual substance use in the past. 'Inebriety' was a term that had encompassed alcohol and other drugs within the same framing applying to both sets of substances but with a particular emphasis on alcohol. 'Addiction', however, was not a combined term and the connection between 'addiction' and 'drug' is demonstrated in the figures. The ascent of addiction occurred against a backdrop of continued use of a mix of terms and common interchange of, for example, 'morphinism', 'morphine habit' or 'morphinomania' within the medical texts surveyed. This was a period of flux in agreed terminology but the general trends—the rise and decline of inebriety and the rise of addiction focussed on drugs other than alcohol—were clear. Through the British Society for the Study of Inebriety and its medical membership, the terminology was 'owned' by a well defined medical group.[18]

In the three other European countries, however, the picture differed. Unlike the UK, none had a substantial tradition of historical research and debate on alcohol, tobacco and other drugs, and so our work was breaking new ground in many ways. In Italy, there was rising interest in specifically alcohol related issues in this period—seven articles between 1860 and 1889, increasing to 45 in the 1890–1909 time span, and finally 71 between 1910 and 1930. Terms also proliferated—including 'alcoholic psychosis', 'alcoholic paranoia', 'pathological drunkenness', and 'delirium tremens'. There was a expansion in the number of terms at the same time as their use was increasing, but the most used concept was 'alcoholism'. Concepts used to characterise other drugs were concentrated at the turn of the nineteenth century (1895–1905) and in the 1920s, but were much more sporadic in their appearance. The terms were divided in a similar way between those concerned with physiological aspects such as 'morphine and cocaine poisoning', and those that deepened the pathological issues, like 'morphinism', 'cocainism' or 'morphinomania'. A major difference between Italy and Britain came in the professional ownership of the issue.[19] In Italy, the experts interested in substance use were part of the school of positivist criminology associated with the work of Cesare Lombroso. In the UK, alcohol and drug issues were dealt with by medical professionals, not criminologists, although like Italy, some of these doctors were influenced by hereditarian ideas.

In Austria, there were further differences. Here it seems that two sets of terminology existed in relation to alcohol and to a lesser extent for other drugs. At first sight the terminology clustered around the words 'alcohol' and 'alcoholism'– with parallel terms 'morphine' and 'morphinism'. At second sight the local terminology—the German dialect used in Austria—proved to be of comparable importance: it clustered around traditional German expressions about the intake of intoxicating substances—'*trinken*' (drink)—and of its main effects—being '*trunken*' (drunken). 'Alcohol' and 'alcoholism', to contemporary understanding, were foreign words and not part of the local terminology (*Ausdrucksweise*). The assumption that the two terminologies indicated more than one addiction concept was supported by the preference of the legal discourse for the German terminology until the present day and by the twofold addiction concept used in contemporary Austrian psychiatry. The final list included names of substances and verbs for intake and was divided between two families or clusters: the international one was based on '*alkohol*' (alcohol), '*alkoholiker*' (alcoholic) and '*alkoholismus*' (alcoholism), the local on '*trinken*' and '*trunken*'. Both included combinations with core words and derivatives such as '*trinker*' (drinker), '*trinksitte*' (drinking customs), '*trinkerrettung*' (salvation of drinker), '*trunkenheit*' (intoxication), '*trunkenbold*' (drunkard) and '*trunksuch*' (ailing due to drinking).

Analysis of the language used in the Austrian articles reinforced the impression of the existence of two terminologies and of more than one addiction concept: the international terminology was linked to a scientific concept of addiction with one main cause—drinking—and with universal (harmful) consequences, which, after the turn of the century, increasingly included hereditary degeneration. The German terminology conceived *trunksucht* (ailing because of drinking) as an incurable secondary disease of a mental disorder and at the same time as the curable consequence of passion. Both types of addiction were loosely united in one concept, but though the first type was increasingly amalgamated with the scientific concept, the latter could neither penetrate nor replace the local concept used by German speaking Austrians.[20]

In Poland, most of the key words used in our search appeared more or less frequently in the whole period under study, though their meaning or range underwent change. 'Alcoholism', 'drunkenness', 'poisoning', (including chronic and acute) and 'inebriety' were the terms most frequently in use. Dipsomania' appeared rather seldom, as did 'habit'. The term '*nałóg*', which linguistically could be a concept close to addiction, was very rare indeed and used as an adjective as well as a noun. The term 'alcoholism' was used increasingly and at the expense of other terms, in particular that of 'inebriety' which, as in the UK, almost disappeared from the medical debate at the beginning of the twentieth century. During this period in Poland, illicit drugs were of secondary importance in the addiction vocabulary. The concept of drug 'addiction' appeared a decade later than the debate on alcoholism—in the 1880s as opposed to the 1870s—instead the literature adopted the similar concepts of *morfinizm* and *kokainizm* as the major terms relating to drug addiction.

In Poland, our more detailed conclusions were restricted to alcohol addiction as this terminology appeared with sufficient frequency. Initially, in the 1860s, 'inebriety' or 'drunkenness' were perceived as a source of mental disorder due to alcohol's poisonous impact on the human brain but these terms evolved to become 'alcoholism'—a mental disease in its own right—towards the end of the nineteenth century. The concept of alcoholism as an artificially induced madness was also elaborated. This 'artificial insanity' could be short-term (acute) as long as the influence of alcohol lasted, or chronic if inebriety persisted to become a permanent state. At the beginning of the twentieth century, the concept of alcoholism changed again from referring only to the mental disease, to cover all the somatic and mental consequences for the affected individual. Later, in particular after Poland regained its independence, these medical overtones were replaced by social concerns. The term 'alcoholism' tended to cover all medical and social consequences, including major social conditions such as poverty and crime. In addition to medical treatment, temperance and prohibition solutions were discussed. But at the same time, alcoholism was increasingly interpreted as an expression of the individual degeneration of alcoholics and their offspring and, therefore, individual, eugenic control became a solution which was seriously considered. Addiction in general was a concept owned mostly by psychiatrists. That situation changed in the twentieth century when public hygiene and social welfare experts joined psychiatrists, paying attention to the social aspects of addiction and seeking solutions in social interventions.[21]

This brief survey shows that the Anglo-American inebriety model was by no means transferable wholesale to our emergent understanding of concepts in selected European countries in this period. Some countries, such as Poland, did use the terminology of inebriety (restricted to alcohol only) but it was not universal elsewhere in our study. This was a period of flux in language with a multiplicity of terms in use, gradually moving towards some degree of greater standardisation by the end of our period. But a country such as Austria, still maintained a localised language in relation to drunkenness as well as the more international terminology of alcoholism and addiction. It would be interesting to see the extent to which this pattern, particularly around the use of terms related to 'drunkenness', was replicated elsewhere. Different professional traditions of ownership were also apparent, most notable the role of forensic scientists and the influence of Lombrosian criminology in Italy. These will be a fruitful lines of future research that we were unable to pursue here.

There were also some factors and issues in common across our study nations. In all countries, this was a period when interest was rising in these topics and alcohol was initially the dominant substance with other drugs emergent as a separate subject of discussion by the turn of the century, gathering pace around the time of the First World War and afterwards. Although individual country traditions remained strong, two significant areas showed similarities. One was the common interest in theories of heredity at the turn of the nineteenth and twentieth centuries: concern about the 'deterioration of the race' seems to have been a cross-national and perhaps Europe-wide phenomenon. In England, the involvement of alcohol as a 'race poison' in the eugenic debate on national deterioration is well known.[22] The same was the case in other European countries. In Italy, the effect of alcoholism on heredity was frequently quoted.[23] There were similar discussions in Poland and Austria. The influence of such eugenic thought is also a partial explanation of what seems to be another commonality—the growing interest in a 'social' view of alcohol issues in the early twentieth century and in the period after the First World War. In several countries, England for example, and Italy as well as in Poland, there were debates between hereditarian, individualistic positions and more social, problem and poverty focused ones. For instance, in 1919, the Polish Deputy Minister for Public Health asserted that alcoholism was a social disease that could only be cured by physicians and social activists working together.[24]

The other, and related, commonality was evidence of an emergent community of knowledge across these European countries. Most country studies indicated that there were cross-national influences by way of scholars citing other international authors, reviews of books and other means. For example, in Italy, one author, Zerboglio, took the work of Krafft-Ebing and Huss as his reference.[25] In England, the work of the German authority Eduard Levinstein on morphine addiction was widely cited. In Poland, the psychiatrist Frydrych was influenced by a journey in Europe and cited the Swedish physician Magnus Huss and the French psychiatrist Bénédict Morel. In-depth discussion of this interest is not possible here since the major focus of our work was quantitative rather than qualitative. But, it appears to relate to the existing European discussion and elaboration of theories of insanity that also utilised these authorities. These pan-European intellectual influences seem to have been just as influential as the expected role of the temperance movement. This was of key importance in some countries, the UK for example, where medical temperance supporters played a leading role in the professional society. Doctors were also involved in the Austrian temperance movement as they were in Italy.

The period 1860–1930 was thus one of great flux across Europe with respect to the concepts used to describe drug and alcohol use. No single concept or concepts appeared to dominate, and though 'alcoholism' was used in all of the countries studied it did not necessarily mean the same thing. Local discourses, such as that around drink and the drinker in Austria, still had a role to play.

Conclusion

The ability to discern similarities and differences between countries over time is something that can only come from cross-national comparative work. To what extent can digitisation help or hamper this kind of endeavour? Where digital sources exist, these can be extremely useful. We found that for the UK, our digital source base allowed us to identify patterns easily, and also to find things that we did not expect—like the temporary decline in the use of the term 'alcoholism'. This kind of research was thus very good at demonstrating change and continuity over time. Making use of digitised journals was, at least in theory, quicker than drawing on traditional paper sources, and certainly was less time consuming for the UK team than for some of our European partners who had to do hand searches and counts. Ironically, digital source research could be particularly valuable in these very places: in the UK we are blessed with an extensive historiography on drugs and alcohol, whereas in many European countries this is not the case. Searching digital sources for the use of key terms and concepts could provide a quick and easy way to generate a narrative of change and continuity over time for topics and places about which little is known. Such research could then provide a springboard to deeper analysis.

Caution, however, should be exercised, as digitisation does not offer a panacea. For our project, the limited availability of digital sources for our European partners made this aspect of the work particularly challenging. It may be that digitisation projects grow in European countries in the coming years, but this will take time, resources and commitment. The limited availability of digital resources in certain countries must not be allowed to hamper the kind of comparative work that is done, or else existing patterns could be reinforced. In the case of drugs and alcohol, for instance, the relative ease in which British and American sources can be accessed could consolidate the Anglo-American bias in the literature. At the same time, the increased availability of digital sources will encourage more researchers to make use of these, often without an awareness of the advantages and disadvantages these present, or of the particular methodological and technological tools one can use to deal with these. For instance, we encountered a number of technical issues that made searching problematic. The differing formats and ways of accessing publications make it hard to adopt a universal research design and the piece-meal approach that develops as a result can further hamper comparative work.

Some of these problems might have been resolved by using text mining tools and other digital analysis software. Text mining, however, also has its pitfalls. For example, it has been argued, using the results of text mining the digitised London Medical Officer of Health reports, that interwar public health was moving away from a focus on 'moral ills' to a less judgmental stance and a greater focus on prevention. The decline in the frequency of the word 'alcoholism' was one result used to make this point.[26] Our research showed that this decline was only temporary. During and after World War Two, alcoholism was established as the dominant concept. This example shows how digital results need to be triangulated with each other but also with traditional historical research and contextualisation. Focusing only on terms and not the context in which they existed both on the page and more broadly risks missing the bigger picture. The digital age may require us to develop new skills and approaches, but it seems likely that we will also need analogue abilities for some years to come.

Acknowledgments

The research leading to these results or outcomes has received funding from the European Union's Seventh Framework Programme (FP7/2007-2013), under Grant Agreement n° 266813 - Addictions and Lifestyle in Contemporary Europe – Reframing Addictions Project (ALICE RAP – www.alicerap.eu). Participant organisations in ALICE RAP can be seen at www.alicerap.eu/about-alice-rap/partners.html.

The views expressed here reflect those of the authors only and the European Union is not liable for any use that may be made of the information contained therein.

Funding

The research leading to these results or outcomes has received funding from the European Union FP7 (FP7/2007-2013), under Grant Agreement n° 266813 - Addictions and Lifestyle in Contemporary Europe – Reframing Addictions Project (ALICE RAP – www.alicerap.eu).

Disclosure Statement

No potential conflict of interest was reported by the authors.

Notes

1. Mussell, "Nineteenth-Century Newspapers in the Digital Age"; Nicholson, "Counting Culture; Or, How to Read Victorian Newspapers from a Distance"; Liddle, "Reflections on 20,000 Victorian Newspapers"; Brake, "Half Full and Half Empty"; Bingham, "The Digitization of Newspaper Archives"; Steel, "Introduction".
2. Nicholson, "The Digital Turn"; Hitchcock, "Confronting the Digital"; Prescott, "I'd Rather Be a Librarian."
3. See http://www.alicerap.eu Accessed 2 September 2016.

4. Hellman et al., *Concepts of Addictive Substances and Behaviours Across Time and Place*; Berridge et al., "Addiction Through the Ages"; Berridge, Mold, and Walke, "From Inebriety to Addiction"; Berridge et al., "Addiction in Europe, 1860s-1960s."

5. Snelders and Pieters, "Speed in the Third Reich"; Snelders, Pieters, and Meijman, "Alcoholism and Heredity in the Medical Sphere"; Blok, "Pampering 'Needle Freaks' or Caring for Chronic Addicts?"; Stephens, *Germans on Drugs*; Padwa, *Social Poison*.

6. Porter, "The Drinking Man's Disease."

7. Levine, "The Discovery of Addiction."

8. Berridge, "Morality and Medical Science"; Harding, *Opiate Addiction Morality and Medicine*.

9. Valverde, "'Slavery from within'"; Valverde, *Diseases of the Will*.

10. Berridge, "The Society for the Study of Addiction."

11. Berridge, Mold, and Walke, "From Inebriety to Addiction"; Moskalewicz and Herczyńska, "The Changing Meaning of Addiction in Polish Medical Literature of the Late Nineteenth Century and Early Twentieth Century"; Eisenbach-Stangl, "Passion and Insanity"; Beccaria and Petrilli, "The Complexity of Addiction."

12. Berridge et al., "Addiction in Europe, 1860s-1960s"; Mold et al., "Concepts of Addiction in Europe in the 1970s and 1980s"

13. Beccaria and Petrilli, "The Complexity of Addiction."

14. Moskalewicz and Herczyńska, "The Changing Meaning of Addiction in Polish Medical Literature of the Late Nineteenth Century and Early Twentieth Century."

15. Eisenbach-Stangl, "Passion and Insanity."

16. Eisenbach-Stangl; Moskalewicz and Herczyńska, "The Changing Meaning of Addiction in Polish Medical Literature of the Late Nineteenth Century and Early Twentieth Century"; Beccaria and Petrilli, "The Complexity of Addiction."

17. This section draws on work published previously in Berridge et al., "Addiction in Europe, 1860s-1960s."

18. Berridge, Mold, and Walke, "From Inebriety to Addiction."

19. Beccaria and Petrilli, "The Complexity of Addiction."

20. Eisenbach-Stangl, "Passion and Insanity."

21. Moskalewicz and Herczyńska, "The Changing Meaning of Addiction in Polish Medical Literature of the Late Nineteenth Century and Early Twentieth Century."

22. Gutzke, "'The Cry of the Children'."

23. Beccaria and Petrilli, "The Complexity of Addiction," 48.

24. Moskalewicz and Herczyńska, "The Changing Meaning of Addiction in Polish Medical Literature of the Late Nineteenth Century and Early Twentieth Century," 77.

25. Beccaria and Petrilli, "The Complexity of Addiction."

26. Seymour and Blaxill, "Adventures in Text Mining with the London MoH Annual Reports."

References

Beccaria, Franca, and Enrico Petrilli. "The Complexity of Addiction: Different Conceptualizations of Alcohol and Drug Addiction(s) among Italian Scholars in the Late 19th and Early 20th Century." *Social History of Alcohol and Drugs* 28, no. 1 (2014): 34–56.

Berridge, Virginia. "Morality and Medical Science: Concepts of Narcotic Addiction in Britain, 1820-1926." *Annals of Science* 36 (1979): 67–85.

Berridge, Virginia. "The Society for the Study of Addiction: Alcohol and Drug Treatment and Control L884-L988." *Addiction* 85, no. 8 (1990): 983–1097.

Berridge, Virginia, Johan Edman, Alex Mold, and Suzanne Taylor. "Addiction Through the Ages: A Review of the Development of Concepts and Ideas About Addiction in European Countries since the Nineteenth Century and the Role of International Organisations in the Process," 2015. http://www.alicerap.eu/about-alice-rap/areas-a-workpackages/area-1-ownership-of-addiction.html.

Berridge, Virginia, Alex Mold, Franca Beccaria, Grazyna Herczyńska, Jacek Moskalewicz, Enrico Petrilli, and Suzanne Taylor. "Addiction in Europe, 1860s-1960s: Concepts and Responses in Italy, Poland, Austria and the United Kingdom." *Contemporary Drug Problems*, forthcoming.

Berridge, Virginia, Alex Mold, and Jennifer Walke. "From Inebriety to Addiction: Terminology and Concepts in the UK, 1860-1930." *Social History of Alcohol and Drugs* 28, no. 1 (2014): 88–106.

Bingham, Adrian. "'The Digitization of Newspaper Archives: Opportunities and Challenges for Historians.'." *Twentieth Century British History* 21, no. 2 (2010): 225–231. doi:10.1093/tcbh/hwq007.

Blok, Gemma. "Pampering 'Needle Freaks' or Caring for Chronic Addicts?: Early Debates on Harm Reduction in Amsterdam." *Social History of Alcohol and Drugs* 22, no. 2 (2008): 243–261.

Brake, Laurel. "Half Full and Half Empty." *Journal of Victorian Culture* 17, no. 2 (June 1, 2012): 222–229. doi:10.1080/13555502.2012.683149.

Eisenbach-Stangl, Irmgard. "Passion and Insanity: A Twofold Concept of Addiction in Austria before World War Two." *Social History of Alcohol and Drugs* 28, no. 1 (2014): 9–33.

Gutzke, David. "'The Cry of the Children': The Edwardian Medical Campaign against Maternal Drinking." *British Journal of Addiction* 79, no. 1 (1984): 71–84.

Harding, Geoffrey. *Opiate Addiction Morality and Medicine: From Moral Illness to Pathological Disease*. Basingstoke: Macmillan, 1988.

Hellman, Matilda, Virginia Berridge, Karen Duke, and Alex Mold. 2016. *Concepts of Addictive Substances and Behaviours Across Time and Place*. Oxford: Oxford University Press.

Hitchcock, Tim. "Confronting the Digital." *Cultural and Social History* 10, no. 1 (March 1, 2013): 9–23. doi:10.2752/147800413X13515292098070.

Levine, Harry Gene. "The Discovery of Addiction: Changing Conceptions of Habitual Drunkenness in America." *Journal of Studies on Alcohol* 39 (1978): 143–174.

Liddle, Dallas. "Reflections on 20,000 Victorian Newspapers: "Distant Reading" The Times Using The Times Digital Archive." *Journal of Victorian Culture* 17, no. 2 (June 1, 2012): 230–237. doi:10.1080/13555502.2012.683151.

Mold, Alex, Franca Beccaria, Virginia Berridge, Irmgard Eisenbach-Stangl, Grazyna Herczyńska, Jacek Moskalewicz, Enrico Petrilli, and Suzanne Taylor. 2016. "Concepts of Addiction in Europe in the 1970s and 1980s: What Does a Long View Tell Us about Drugs, Alcohol and Tobacco?" In *Concepts of Addictive Substances and Behaviours Across Time and Place*, edited by Matilda Hellman, Virginia Berridge, Karen Duke, and Alex Mold, 15–31. Oxford: Oxford University Press.

Moskalewicz, Jacek, and Grazyna Herczyńska. "The Changing Meaning of Addiction in Polish Medical Literature of the Late Nineteenth Century and Early Twentieth Century." *Social History of Alcohol and Drugs* 28, no. 1 (2014): 57–87.

Mussell, James. "Nineteenth-Century Newspapers in the Digital Age." *Journal of Victorian Culture* 17, no. 2 (June 1, 2012): 221–221. doi:10.1080/13555502.2012.683147.

Nicholson, Bob. "The Digital Turn." *Media History* 19, no. 1 (February 1, 2013): 59–73. doi:10.1080/13688804.2012.752963.

Nicholson, Bob. "Counting Culture; or, How to Read Victorian Newspapers from a Distance." *Journal of Victorian Culture* 17, no. 2 (June 1, 2012): 238–246. doi:10.1080/13555502.2012.683331.

Padwa, Howard. *Social Poison: The Culture and Politics of Opiate Control in Britain and France, 1821-1926.* 1st ed. Baltimore: Johns Hopkins University Press, 2012.

Porter, Roy. "The Drinking Man's Disease: The Pre History of Alcoholism in Georgian Britain." *British Journal of Addiction* 80 (1985): 385–396.

Prescott, Andrew. "I'd Rather Be a Librarian." *Cultural and Social History* 11, no. 3 (September 1, 2014): 335–341. doi:10.2752/147800414X13983595303192.

Seymour, Jane, and Luke Blaxill. "Adventures in Text Mining with the London MoH Annual Reports: Towards an Alternative History of Inter War Public Health." presented at the London Health Histories, Wellcome Trust, London, June 17, 2016. http://blog.wellcomelibrary.org/2016/05/london-health-histories-a-workshop/.

Snelders, Stephen, and Toine Pieters. "Speed in the Third Reich: Metamphetamine (Pervitin) Use and a Drug History From Below." *Social History of Medicine* 24, no. 3 (December 1, 2011): 686–699. doi:10.1093/shm/hkq101.

Snelders, Stephen, Toine Pieters, and Frans Meijman. "Alcoholism and Heredity in the Medical Sphere: The Netherlands 1850-1900." *Social History of Alcohol and Drugs* 22, no. 2 (2008): 130–143.

Steel, John. "Introduction." *Media History* 20, no. 1 (January 2, 2014): 1–3. doi:10.1080/13688804.2013.872410.

Stephens, Robert P. *Germans on Drugs: The Complications of Modernization in Hamburg.* Ann Arbor: University of Michigan Press, 2007.

Valverde, Mariana. "'Slavery from within': The Invention of Alcoholism and the Question of Free Will." *Social History* 22, no. 3 (1997): 251–268.

Valverde, Mariana. *Diseases of the Will: Alcohol and the Dilemmas of Freedom.* Cambridge: Cambridge University Press, 1998.

Index

Page numbers in **bold** refer to tables and in *italics* to figures.